HISTORY OF MEDICINE

Tim Hall
with illustrations by
Sir Quentin Blake

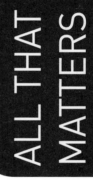

ALL THAT MATTERS

ALL THAT MATTERS

First published in Great Britain in 2013 by Hodder & Stoughton. An Hachette UK company.

First published in US in 2013 by The McGraw-Hill Companies, Inc.

This edition published 2013

British Library Cataloguing in Publication Data: a catalogue record for this title is available from the British Library.

Library of Congress Catalog Card Number: on file.

10 9 8 7 6 5 4 3 2 1

The publisher has used its best endeavours to ensure that any website addresses referred to in this book are correct and active at the time of going to press. However, the publisher and the author have no responsibility for the websites and can make no guarantee that a site will remain live or that the content will remain relevant, decent or appropriate.

The publisher has made every effort to mark as such all words which it believes to be trademarks. The publisher should also like to make it clear that the presence of a word in the book, whether marked or unmarked, in no way affects its legal status as a trademark.

Every reasonable effort has been made by the publisher to trace the copyright holders of material in this book. Any errors or omissions should be notified in writing to the publisher, who will endeavour to rectify the situation for any reprints and future editions.

Typeset by Cenveo® Publisher Services.

Printed and bound in Great Britain by CPI Group (UK) Ltd., Croydon, CR0 4YY.

Hodder & Stoughton policy is to use papers that are natural, renewable and recyclable products and made from wood grown in sustainable forests. The logging and manufacturing processes are expected to conform to the environmental regulations of the country of origin.

Hodder & Stoughton Ltd

338 Euston Road

London NW1 3BH

www.hodder.co.uk

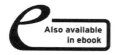

Contents

With enormous thanks to Sir Quentin Blake for his gift of original illustrations to Tim Hall for this book.

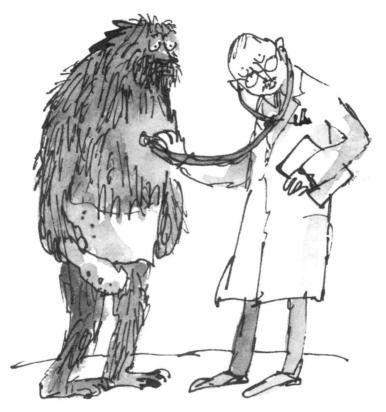

Preface

If a lady dinosaur (anywhere from her dinosaur period 230 to 65 million years ago) were somehow resurrected, transplanted into our world, ushered into a modern maternity unit (she might need shrinking a little, depending upon her species), and able to talk to us, she would probably – once overcoming her initial surprise at all that – declare that maternity care is instinctively the same as it was in her day.

For as long as humans have evolved they have sought ways to parry death, disease and discomfort. Orang-utans wash the faces of their young at riverbanks. Howler monkeys wipe bloodied wounds with wet leaves. The most primitive animals know that rest after injury helps healing, and nurturing their young provides optimum temperature and nutrition for survival, just as a neonatal unit's incubator supports a sick baby.

Dinosaurs were doubtless the same.

In October 1984 nine Aboriginal people were discovered in Western Australia's vast Gibson Desert. They were naked, and had never seen a white person before. They were living a nomadic lifestyle, something humans had done for most of their history.

Ancestors we might recognize as human-like emerged 6-10 million years ago. Almost 2 million years ago they had become upright *Homo erectus*, making tools and fire and eventually learning to speak. Around 200,000 to 150,000 years ago they looked much like you and me, *Homo sapiens*. They led harsh, brief lives, but in small, roving groups they evaded the plagues of infections that thrive on population density. Food came from hunting and gathering, rather than from domesticated animals and cultivated crops, reservoirs for micro-organisms. And since wild food supplies were soon exhausted, humans seldom stayed anywhere long enough to contaminate local water sources.

October 1984 was monumentally sobering, a meeting of who we are now and who we once were. And immediately, the last nomadic people developed our diseases.

Early humans viewed death supernaturally. Disease arose by projecting morbid material into the body (as with Aboriginal bone-pointing, or a snake-bite arranged by a sorcerer) or by abstracting the soul from the body.

Folk medicine, for want of a better term, has indistinct origins. Massage was thought to dispel unwanted spirits. The notion of disease transference through touch pervades history. In later times, hangmen would receive money for allowing the sick to touch the executed. In Lancashire the cure for warts was touching a pebble. In Cumberland the remedy for whooping cough was inserting the head of freshly caught fish in the affected child's mouth, returning it to the river to take the 'whoop' with it. Swimming through a hole in a popular rock in Scotland's River Dee was thought to cure infertility.

Charms, amulets and talismans have also endured from time immemorial. Until relatively recently it was not uncommon to keep a potato in the pocket to ease arthritis. A hare's forefoot cured many ills, as did a coffin's nail. A bezoar hairball from a goat's stomach warded off poisons. There was the power of 'sympathy', too – the hair of a dog that bit you could also be applied to cure you.

In the mid-nineteenth century, anthropologists began to look at prehistoric skulls with greater curiosity. Holes in excavated skulls were known to be commonplace, but always assumed to be a result of weaponry. Many such skulls were unearthed in France, some 5,000 years old, and in some burial chambers most skulls contained artificial holes. One turned up near the future Hammersmith Bridge in London; others near the coast in Dorset. And then a writer in *The Lancet* in 1888 reported that he had found evidence of the practice of cutting holes in skulls in living humans – trepanning, as it was called – still extant near the Caspian Sea. Trepanning was originally thought to remove ill-mannered loitering spirits, but was later used on head injuries. While it doubtless compounded the injury, evidence of skull healing reveals that many subjected to trepanning lived for many more years.

We could dwell endlessly on these endless practices, with prehistoric roots. But we must return to that fluid time on Earth when prehistory started to dissolve into periods we can more tangibly date.

The Ages of Antiquity and Darkness

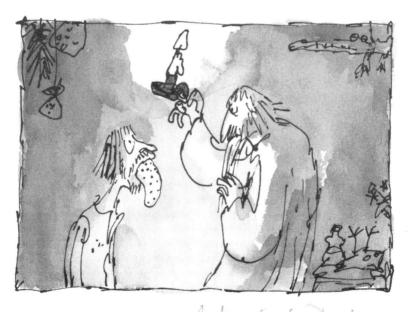

1

The Age of Ice
and Caves

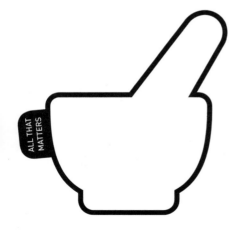

ALL THAT
MATTERS

▶ Caves to 'civilization'

Perhaps the most arresting object in the British Museum is a delicate carving from a mammoth tusk of two swimming reindeer, 13,000 years old. Fashioned by a sculptor who knew animal anatomy well (if humans could hunt they could survive), it also provides evidence of a human brain adapted to imagination and art. Indeed the earliest known cave art, 50,000 years old, in Arnhem Land, Australia, points to a human brain shifting from one almost exclusively engaged in survival to one developing social tendencies.

The shift from human tool-maker to artist, perhaps imperative in long, harsh winters, tells us something about the way the world was beginning to be perceived. Animal art in paintings, carvings and jewellery suggests social bonding. Against the perils of life, humans in social groups were no longer driven solely to survive, but to share their world in more eloquent ways. With this came a regard for morbidity and mortality not just for oneself, but also for others, and a desire to protect each other from threats. That, in the most rudimentary yet startlingly clear terms, is what a system of health and social welfare is all about.

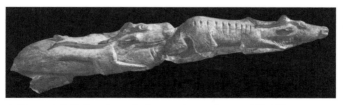

▲ Figure 1.1 Swimming reindeer sculpture (around 13,000 years old), carved from mammoth tusk, found at Montastruc, central France. British Museum.

▶ Ice to agriculture

In the winter of 1850 a storm of such fury swept through Scotland's Orkney Islands that inhabitants of one coastal village awoke to find evidence of human life that could be traced back 5,000 years. Skara Brae, exposed when the beach's sand was swept away, is an archaeological site older than the pyramids, remarkable not so much in its stone dwellings but in the sophisticated way its people lived. Each house has near identical fittings (suggesting egalitarianism): a central hearth and adjacent stone box beds that would have been packed with heather; a dresser with a seat; alcoves and shelves; locking doors; water tanks; and systems of plumbing and drainage to keep everyone dry. Inhabitants had jewellery and pottery, grew crops, harvested fish, and kept livestock. They liked dogs. They burned seaweed, a rather unsatisfying fuel, but one thing lacking was trees – something of enormous satisfaction to historians, for nothing would have remained of Skara Brae had it been constructed from wood.

Not that Skara Brae was instantly of interest. The site was popular with local youths for partying and pillaging, and, though less damaging archaeologically, promiscuity, but when in 1924 a storm swept part of a dwelling into the sea it was decided to preserve the site formally.

Vere Gordon Childe was not a trained archaeologist – few people were at that time – having read Classics and Philosophy in his native Australia before arriving in Oxford in 1914, largely to read and think. Childe had an inordinate preference for library studies over fieldwork, his contemplations making him an authority on the lives of prehistoric people. He was a master of ancient texts and languages, and a dab hand in many unlikely skills such as long division in Roman numerals. In 1927 he was appointed to the new post of Abercrombie

Professor of Prehistoric Archaeology at the University of Edinburgh, the institution that sent its reluctant appointee to examine Skara Brae.

Childe was, by all accounts, a man with many shortcomings as well as rather odd spectacles, but when eventually prised from his library to Skara Brae he had indubitably the greatest idea in the history of archaeology. Childe conceptualized the most momentous event in human history, that threshold between 'prehistory' and 'civilization', and called it the Neolithic Revolution.

The development of communities with farming and irrigation, and all the bits of society referred to as 'civilization', began after the Ice Age. For most of their history, humans did very little but survive. And then something happened. Scientists cannot tell us why, only what, when and where, but perhaps pivotal was the weather. Approximately 12,000 years ago the Earth warmed, plunging back to icy times for about a thousand years, before warming rapidly again to stay that way since. All human 'advances' have occurred in this brief spell since. As Sir William Osler commented in his *Evolution of Modern Medicine* lectures at Yale in 1913, 'Civilization is but a filmy fringe on the history of man'; historian Ronald Wright says in his *A Short History of Progress*, 'The greatest wonder of the ancient world is how recent it all is. No city or monument is much more than 5000 years old. Only about seventy lifetimes, of seventy years, have been lived end to end since civilization began. Its entire run occupies a mere 0.2 percent of the two and a half million years since our first ancestor sharpened a stone.'

Notable about the Neolithic Revolution, as well as it happening at all, is that it happened independently all over the earth, albeit at different times. Unknown to one another, people did the same thing everywhere. Farming appeared in the

Middle East, Africa, China, the Andes and the Amazon. Cities sprouted in Mesopotamia, Egypt, China, India and Central America, and Wright's observation is telling: 'When Cortes landed in Mexico he found roads, canals, cities, palaces, schools, law courts, markets, irrigation works, kings, priests, temples, peasants, artisans, armies, astronomers, merchants, sports, theatre, art, music, and books. High civilization, differing in detail but alike in essentials, had evolved independently on both sides of the earth.'

Farming started in the Levant – the intersection of western Asia, the eastern Mediterranean and northeast Africa – perhaps 10,000 years ago (8000 BC). The melted ice left lush savannah (now mostly Saharan desert) with gazelles, giraffes, zebras, elephants and wild cattle – happy hunting ground for nomads. Then around 6000 BC rains diminished, food supplies dwindled, and cows were the most facilitating animals to herd and eat. By now farming had reached the Nile valley and southern Europe. It began a little later in China and later still in the Americas, around 4000 BC.

Converting grasses into food was hard work, and unexpected (grass is not an obvious human foodstuff). Yet across the world grass came under scrutiny by humans: wheat and barley in the Middle East, millet in northern China and rice further south.

Cows were fairly agreeable animals, and seemingly in agreement with (or at least irresistant to) the arrangement to be widely herded. By 7000 BC sheep and goats were domesticated. By 5000 BC pigs were being reared. Half a millennium later horses were domesticated on Eurasian steppes, people having lived with animals for thousands of years before it occurred to anyone to try them with a plough. Dogs were domesticated as far as England, Siberia and North America. It isn't known when we started keeping chickens.

Nothing we take for granted today – language and writing, art and architecture, towns and cities, music and literature, commerce and industry, law and government, healthcare and medicine – would be possible without agriculture. Once we farmed, we had enough food, and enough time, to do more than hunting.

▶ Distant history to disease

For the first few million years of their existence humans lived in scattered groups of maybe 50 to 100 individuals, such low numbers parrying the pathogens that thrive on population density.

Civilization brought food and safety, but at a price. Jaw abscesses came from teeth shattered by fragments of stone used for grinding grain. Nomads had eaten more protein and vitamins, and taken higher calorific intake, than settled people with plainer diets who succumbed to dietary insufficiencies like pellagra, marasmus and kwashiorkor. But the over-arching threat brought by agriculture and animal husbandry was infection.

Bacteria, viruses, worms and parasites, and intermediate hosts for many micro-organisms – fleas, mosquitoes, ticks and lice – began to co-exist, locked in evolutionary struggles for survival with humans. Adaptation allowed microbes to jump species and reside comfortably – if uncomfortably to their newfound hosts – in humans. Cattle spread tuberculosis and smallpox. Pigs and ducks passed on influenzas. Horses provided the common cold. And dogs gave us measles, arising from canine distemper. Cholera, polio, typhoid, hepatitis, whooping cough and diphtheria organisms found human water supplies irresistible. Bacteria, fungi, rodent excrement and insects settled nicely into granaries. Worms started to squirm and squat in humans, too: roundworms found their way from pigs to humans; the notoriously lengthy hookworms found the human gut an ideal place to regale themselves; and filarial worms brought, as well as unenviable river blindness, the alarmingly affecting and disarmingly disfiguring elephantiasis.

Between 4000 BC and 2000 BC the first urban civilizations arose in the 'Fertile Crescent' of Mesopotamia (now Iraq) between the Euphrates and Tigris rivers, Egypt's Nile delta, the Indus valley in Pakistan and along the Yellow and Yangtze rivers in China. These rivers ebbed and flowed seasonally, and humans built dams to store water in reservoirs and ditches to water fields in dry seasons. Wherever agriculture relied on irrigation, watery fields harboured worms that could live partly submerged and partly exploring humans after burrowing into feet (symptoms of schistosomiasis depend upon the journey the worm thereafter fancies).

Stagnant water-filled furrows also proved perfect breeding grounds for a vector whose disease has remained a globally insurmountable cause of death and disease – the female *Anopheles* mosquito, and her protozoan malarial parasite *Plasmodium*. The worst kind, *Plasmodium falciparum*, spends its developing life, after mosquito bite injection, in the human liver and blood, parasitizing and destroying cells and provoking the deadly black-water fever and cerebral malaria. Moving from Africa to the Middle East, India, south China and the New World via shipping, malaria continues its global advance as global warming expands mosquito breeding grounds. Darwinian adaptations have often done their bit to keep pace. The sickle cell trait in black Africans affords protection against one type of malaria, *Plasmodium vivax*. Unhappily some genetic mutations result in full-blown sickle cell disease, with unhappier consequences than the perils of vivax malaria. And, ironically, the trait itself would make black Africans ideal for slave plantations in the New World.

In short, disease settled happily in settled humans, and has never gone away.

2

The Age of
Antiquity (I)

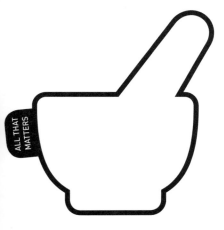

ALL THAT
MATTERS

▶ Mesopotamia and medicine most shadowy

The first large civilization appeared around 4000 BC in Mesopotamia: the Sumerian city Ur. Sumerians had bathrooms, wheeled vehicles and tools. They wrote on clay tablets. They practised medicine, but of it we know little. Around 2000 BC Mesopotamia passed to the southern Babylonians and northern Assyrians. A Babylonian king drew up the oldest known code of law, including medical practice.

▶ Egypt and medicine most ancient

In 1900 a member of the Egypt Exploration Society excavated a grave in Abydos in southern Egypt and noted, among its contents, a 'stand of 4 clay cows'. Many of us, contemplating ancient Egypt, might imagine ourselves entering Tutankhamun's tomb with awe and trepidation, arrested by its treasures and the spectre of its curse. Four small cows might prepossess us least. It was certainly the last item on the excavator's list, ranking after 'a male body', a 'baton of painted clay', a 'small red pottery box' and the 'legs of a small animal'.

The cows were fashioned from Nile river clay, equivalent to modern toy farm animals, and traces of paint still linger. They look somewhat different from modern cows, all now of Asian descent; ancient Egypt's came from Africa.

The cows, 5,500 years old, stand today in the British Museum. They were made long after humans began domesticating cattle, and thus long after humans started encountering zoonotic disease – disease acquired from animals – but Egypt was still embryonic. Cows then were not milked; it would be millennia before human genes adapted to milk's lactose. But along the Nile valley, cows had long been sources of meat, and security, and they transformed human existence.

In this painstakingly selective account of medicine's history, it seems amiss to observe so fleetingly a civilization that would endure longer than any other, to skirt so wilfully around life in its kingdoms. Yet these little cows doubtless represent the double-edged sword of human advance and disease susceptibility more than any of the Egypt, with its pharaohs and pyramids, yet to come. It would be more than 2,000 years before Tutankhamun's short life, by which time Egyptians had long realized a reliance on cows that is impossible to overstate. Without cows, civilizations might not have survived at all.

Egypt endured from 3500 BC, around the time our little cows were made, for three millennia. Although the relics are bold, little was known about Egyptian life until the discovery in Alexandria in 1799 of the Rosetta Stone, the text of which

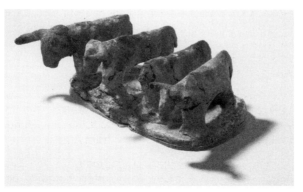

▲ Figure 2.1 Egyptian clay model of cattle. From el-Amra, Egypt, Predynastic, Naqada I period, around 3500 BC. British Museum.

allowed interpreters to decipher Egyptian hieroglyphics. And so we know that in 3100 BC Menes united upper and lower Egypt and created Memphis, and that ancient Egyptians would go on to experience three kingdoms and 31 dynasties without any notion of Elvis Aaron Presley and the music genres with which the name of its first city would later become associated.

More sedentary life brought diverse societal roles, and hierarchy. Pyramids were tombs for the dead, the earliest for pharaohs, containing objects needed in an afterlife, and it was crucial that bodies be preserved: embalmed or 'mummified'. The earliest intact mummy dates from around 3400 BC, Mummy 32751 in the British Museum, named 'Ginger' for his hair colour (until the practice of naming mummies was deemed insensitive); mummification may not have been intended, since he appears to have been mummified by desert sand. Embalmers used salts to remove body moisture, a complicated process taking months, and to prevent decomposition internal organs were removed. Lungs, stomach, liver and intestines were plopped into jars and placed close to the body, alongside less 'vital' possessions and potions.

Mummified Egyptian remains are so delicate that they may crumble if physically examined. Modern radiology and molecular analysis allows scientists, without tampering, to identify diseases still with us today such as arthritis, osteomyelitis and tuberculosis. The mummy of Hornedjitef, a high-ranking priest who died around 240 BC, reveals exactly this. More than 2,000 years earlier Imhotep, physician and architect, as well as designing Egypt's first burial place – the Step Pyramid at Saqqara – advised treatment on over 200 diseases (of no benefit, one must concede, to Hornedjitef). In ancient Egypt the physician was one type of healer, amid sorcerers and priests. One physician, Iri, was the pharaoh's enema expert; another, Peseshet, a female physician. Imhotep was the most famous, possibly because his assertions were written down.

Egypt was rich in agriculture but poor in wine, timber and precious stones. Trade with other peoples eventually became alluring. As did war. So often through history disease has been delivered through merchants and mariners exchanging novel infections as well as wares. For Egypt marauding attack added to the disquiet of disease, firstly from the mysterious eastern Mediterranean 'sea-peoples', and later invasion by the Assyrians and Persians and finally by Alexander the Great in 332 BC, when Greece would be the mightiest empire in the world.

▶ India and China and medicine more philosophical

Before considering Greece, we should step momentarily eastwards.

In the first millennium BC, the Atharvaveda was the first Indian medical text and Ayurveda, traditional Indian medicine, emerged comprising the Suśruta and Charaka. Malaria was associated with mosquitoes, plague with dead rats. Medicinal plants were commonplace. But in surgery Indian medicine excelled, in procedures bold and distinctive. Fractures were set with bamboo splints. Cataracts were peeled. And of peculiar interest was rhinoplasty, often needed because adulterers' noses were removed. A tree leaf was cut to shape and size, modelling the new nose, and corresponding cheek or forehead skin cut and sutured in position.

Acupuncture may have been used around 700 BC. Moxibustion, in which the combustible mugwort herb was ignited on skin, must have demanded considerable self-control on the part of the patient. Ancient Chinese medicine was, if not always effective, pioneeringly diverse. Inoculation against smallpox was practised, dried crusts from a smallpox patient insufflated into the nose. 'Cretins' (suffering from hypothyroidism) were fed on sheep thyroid glands. Cannabis was used for anaesthesia.

Traditional Chinese medicine is steeped in philosophy. *Yin* and *Yang* symbolize two complementary sides of every phenomenon in the universe, including the body, such as fire and water. Being 'healthy' requires *Yin* and *Yang* balance. Disequilibrium could cause fieriness and fever, or fluid accumulation. The 'Five Elements' philosophy ascribes elements to organs: wood, liver; water, kidney; fire, heart; earth, spleen; metal, lung. Disease in one organ adversely affects another, this interdependence requiring a holistic approach to patients. The *Yellow Emperor's Inner Canon*, compiled in the last few centuries BC, is one of the earliest books incorporating these philosophies.

Chinese medicine endured, oddly, despite its lack of rationality.

Rationality, though, was something the Greeks would make their own.

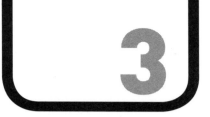

3

The Age of
Antiquity (II)

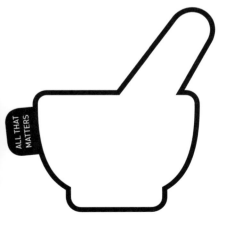

ALL THAT
MATTERS

▶ Greece and medicine more rational

One of the greatest love stories of the ancient world involved Seleucus I, king of Syria (358-280 BC), whose whim in mature years was to marry a rather younger woman, Stratonice. Unhappily Antiochus, Seleucus's son by his first wife, fell madly in love with his stepmother Stratonice. 'Mindful of the immorality of the passion that burned in him', penned Roman historian Valerius Maximus, and tormented by 'utmost desire and deepest shame', Antiochus retreated into silence. He wasted away with such alarming alacrity that court physicians decided to summon a medical eminence, Erasistratus. Erasistratus (c. 304–250 BC) practised in Egypt's Alexandria, the erudite hub of the Hellenic world, where, with fellow physician Herophilus (c. 330–260 BC), he founded a school of anatomy. Erasistratus allegedly first described the heart's valves, and appears to have concluded that the heart was not the seat of sentience, and love, but merely a pump. He distinguished arteries from veins, although he believed arteries were full of air carrying the vital spirit 'pneuma'. He seemed to appreciate that invisible particles were essential body elements, believing these to be vitalized by the pneuma that also pervaded nerves, and that nerves were networks transducing the brain's spirit. He made some distinction between sensory and motor nerves, and described the cerebrum and cerebellum. But Erasistratus's greatest achievement, perhaps, was his description of a condition that still today has no apter term, no better physiological understanding and no easy treatment: lovesickness.

Erasistratus promptly diagnosed Antiochus's illness by taking his pulse. He noted that each time Stratonice came within sight of his patient, his patient's pulse hastened, his voice faltered and he would blush and sweat. None of this occurred in the presence of other women.

It was one of those happy situations where, of sorts, everybody won. Erasistratus deliberated then decided upon a quiet word with the king, who yielded his wife. Seleucus regained a son. Antiochus gained a wife. Stratonice, by most accounts, gained her preference. And Erasistratus became royal physician.

If, in this painstakingly selective narrative of medicine's history, it seems remiss to dismiss so much of Egypt, then it seems frankly illicit to graze so scantily in the fields of Greece, and our story about lovesickness might seem wastefully discursive. Yet if there is one defining legacy of the Greeks – and they left us many – then it is their desire to understand the world rationally, and reflect it aesthetically. They appreciated love, for both their people and their world. Greece provided rich pastures for nurturing medicine, for the Greeks were humanist, curious and 'refined'. Much of our language, art, architecture, philosophy, education, politics, science and medicine traces back to ancient Greece, considered the foundation of Western civilization (somewhat surprising since Greece was not a unified state but a collection of peoples scattered around the Mediterranean). Ancient Greece may or may not – historians argue – include the Minoan and Mycenaean civilizations and the tales of Troy and the Trojan War told by Homer; most historians are tranquil taking ancient Greece from the first Olympic Games and dividing it into four periods: Archaic (750–500 BC), Classical (500–323 BC), Hellenistic (323–146 BC) and Roman (146 BC–330 AD).

Archaic Greece was still in the Orient's mythological breeze, steeped in legend. Apollo was born on Delos, an island in azure sea raised by Zeus from the seabed. Apollo left for Delphi, site of the famous Oracle of wisdom (although that oracle did once advise that a lake which inhabitants of a town wanted to drain – they felt it to be, doubtless correct, a source of malaria – ought be undisturbed). The supernatural pervaded early Greek medicine, as it had with Egyptians, although in Greece disease was attributable to gods, not demons. In Homer's *Iliad,* Apollo destroys Greece's army, besieging Troy, with a plague. In Hesiod's *Works and Days*, it is Zeus who sends plagues and famines. Pandora's Box, immortalized in *Works and Days*, was in fact a jar containing all evils of the world. When Prometheus stole fire from heaven, Zeus took vengeance by presenting the edgily seductive Pandora to Prometheus's brother. But Pandora, impelled by curiosity, opened the jar and evil escaped and spread across the earth. She hastened to close it, but all that could be contained was one thing at the bottom, an angel of Hope. To 'open Pandora's box' now means to unleash irrevocable problems. It was the Greek gods who, as well as unleashing plagues, effected cures, especially in Asclepian temples.

Asclepius, god of healing, son of Apollo, is often depicted with his daughters Hygeia (health) and Panacea (cure-all), and sons who became the first physicians (Asclepiads). By 200 BC all cities would have healing temples with sleeping chambers where the sick, incubated in visionary dreams in which Asclepius advised, received cures. The best known was on the island of Cos, reputedly Hippocrates' birthplace.

Classical Greece was first dominated by Athens, then displaced by Sparta before power shifted to Thebes and finally Macedon. Two major wars shaped the Classical world: the Persian Wars, in which Greece's sea-bound cities revolted from Persia (Iran), and the Peloponnesian War between Athens and Sparta, which would later reunite. It is in Classical Greece that we find Hippocrates.

In a shift from sacred to secular thinking, Hippocratic doctors professed natural causes for disease and sought natural healing, acting in complement to gods in whom they still believed. Hippocrates himself is a misty figure. He may have lived 460–377 BC, a touch earlier than Aristotle, and most tales of him are probably untrue. One of the more challenging endeavours if you are incarcerated in prison for 20 years without resource, even with mental acuity impressive, memory perfectly agile, is to write a comprehensive treatise. Hippocrates, if this one extract of his life is to be believed, could not have written the 60 or so volumes of the *Hippocratic Corpus*. He probably didn't cure a Macedonian king of lovesickness. Or burn down a temple. But fancifully he did, when philosopher Democritus was presented to him as mad (because Democritus laughed at everything), diagnose merely a happy disposition.

Hippocratic medicine is more of a historical construct, the *Corpus* perhaps no more penned by Hippocrates than *Iliad* by Homer but Hippocratic medicine, explaining health and disease in terms of 'humours', dominated the Classical world. The body's rhythms were thought to be determined by four humours or fluids, health or illness resulting from how these equilibrated. Blood, red, was for vitality. Choler or bile, yellow, was for digestion. Phlegm was a lubricant and coolant, comprising all colourless secretions including snot, sweat and tears, and was most evident in illness. Black bile was a constant source of unrest; it coloured skin, urine and stool, and provoked melancholy. The humours provoked all manifestations of health and illness. Blood made the body hot and wet, choler hot and dry, phlegm cold and wet, and black bile cold and dry. Parallels were drawn with the natural world and seasons. Blood was like air, choler like fire, phlegm like water and black bile like the earth. Cold and wet, winter was when people developed phlegm and chills. The humours dictated physique and persona, too. Phlegmatics were fat, cholerics thin. Bloody people were energetic but prone to temper and impulse. Cholerics were quick to anger. The coolness of phlegmatics impelled them to laziness. Those bent towards black bile saw the world darkly, and were ponderous and suspicious.

Humoral medicine would persist for almost two millennia. With four variables creating infinite permutations as to the degree a body was in or out of balance, the theory was difficult to disprove. And the appetite for a treatment was satiated by the lure of cure. Practitioners could recommend diets, exercises or bloodletting to recalibrate a humour in deficit or surfeit. Snakes, harmless varieties, were popularized by the Greeks who felt they aided harmony of the humours by licking eyes and wounds.

Hippocratic medicine had two major difficulties. The first was that it was without scientific foundation: the Greeks knew little anatomy or physiology other than that gleaned from animals, for human dissection was deemed disrespectful and virtually forbidden. The second, consequent upon the first, was that it was not exactly effective. But Hippocratic doctors did lay a guiding principle that endures today: the 'first rule of medicine, to do no harm'.

As Greece traded and warred with other worlds, one region's tamed disease was another's epidemic. Just as pestilences had plagued Egypt, the plague in 430 BC in Athens proved devastating. Historian Thucydides recounted 'discharges of bile of every kind', and pustules of such severity that sufferers 'could not bear clothing or linen even of the very lightest description; or indeed to be otherwise than stark naked'. It was possibly bubonic plague, possibly smallpox, possibly something else, even chickenpox, for diseases now considered mild such as chickenpox once killed or immunized with ferocity in regions virgin to exposure until microbes died out for lack of hosts. We don't know what it was, but it spelled the end of the ascendency of Athens.

Epidemics and wars, however, did not quell Greece's desire to develop a society that valued humanity – the Romans would value conquest more – and in such a society medicine was revered. That said, it would be difficult to find a hospital in ancient Greece, more so a surgeon. The *Corpus* included a wounds treatise that advised realigning fractures, advocated extracting nasal polyps and admired cautery – red hot iron to sear and seal flesh – on haemorrhoids (which cannot have invoked in patients the sense that symptoms would soon be assuaged). But the Greeks admonished use of the knife. They neither ligatured wounds, nor knew much anatomy. They were, by and large, physicians who sat with patients in one-to-one consultations, deliberating over the kilter of the humours.

But importantly, Classical Greeks introduced rational medicine, even if it lacked scientific rigour, in which diseases had physical causes. Philosophers and scientists began to reject mythical explanations of their world. Pythagoras explained it arithmetically (though his pupil, Empedocles, clearly still allied to mythological worlds, leapt into the crater of Mount Etna that he might become a god). Socrates sought ethical and political answers. Plato considered alternatives to those things immediately perceived. His pupil Aristotle was analytical, pondering big questions about the natural world: why plants germinate and animals are born, and why these grow and die; why seasons occurred; and why apples fell from trees and discoloured. Euclid fancied things geometric. Archimedes' penchant was mechanics. Greek art and architecture reflected these things in geometry, proportion, balance and calm. Sophocles penned poetry. Herodotus told history, and Strabo gave us geography. Phidius built the Parthenon, Praxiteles lovely statues. These Greeks sought perfection. Plastic surgeons today still fashion noses on classical aesthetics.

And so it was, in this shift from 'supernatural' to 'natural' thinking, that medicine developed rationality. The *Corpus*'s treatises are virtually free from magic. In one, *Sacred Disease,* the author asserts a natural cause for epilepsy, and though attributed to phlegm blocking passages from the brain, the explanation was far more logical than evil spirits residing in the brain, a notion that would return to medicine in darker times ahead.

But, for a while at least, the world could bask in expanding reverence for logic.

▶ Greece and medicine most refined

By the Hellenistic period – beginning with Alexander's death and ending with Roman conquest – Greece had expanded into the near and middle east, but its scholarly and artistic epoch was to fade. Alexandrian medicine, dominating Hellenistic Greece, had inherited the dread of corpses and taboos about dissection, but in the third century BC the notable – one must speculate if noble – Herophilus started dissecting human cadavers (some say human vivisection of slaves and criminals) publicly. A contemporary of Erasistratus, whom we last met contemplating the bittersweet sickness and joyousness of love, Herophilus named the prostate and duodenum ('twelve fingers' in length) and established that arteries were filled with blood, much to the consternation of his audiences. But most indelicate, to his audiences at least, yet most delicate in precision, Herophilus dissected entire nervous systems and demonstrated how these connected to the brain. The brain was the seat of the soul, of intelligence and emotion, and to show that it was nerves, not blood vessels, that conveyed the soul's impulses, may have first perturbed Erasistratus, whose authority on the science of emotion was second to none. But Erasistratus would come to the conviction, too, that the brain and nervous system governed thoughts and actions, and would spend much of his life making dissection spectacular art.

We know little of the Medical School of Alexandria, other than of Herophilus and Erasistratus, and Alexandria (once seat of the world's largest library and a lighthouse that was one of the Seven Wonders of the Ancient World) would be extinguished by Rome. But medicine in Rome, if nothing else, would remain in the hands of the Greeks.

Various sects arose in Graeco-Roman times. Pneumatists attributed just about every human condition to the airy spirit. Rationalists expounded natural philosophy ('science'). Empiricists emphasized visible symptoms. And methodists enjoyed the simple premise that disease depended on the tenseness or laxity of the body, happily rejecting all other notions. But in the second century AD, a physician would emerge, self-appointed, self-important and bold, with natural philosophical leaning, whose legacy would stand for a millennium and a half. Galen (129–c. 216) was a master of dissection: not of humans, admittedly, but in dissecting dogs, pigs, sheep and goats there was no other, and he once deftly dissected an elephant. These animal surrogates would be sources of error, for Galen asserted that human hearts had three ventricles and livers five lobes, but nobody knew better to challenge him, or would have tried. Galen regarded colleagues as blustering buffoons, and patients possibly with contempt. He hid the latter well: patient trust, he argued, was won through good bedside manner. The former he made no attempt to conceal. The physician, he argued, should be master of logic (the art of thinking), physics (the science of nature) and ethics (the rule of action). That he considered himself unrivalled in these was evident in his writing: 'It is I, and I alone, who have revealed the true path of medicine. It must be admitted that Hippocrates already staked out this path ... he prepared the way, but I have made it passable.'

In 162, Galen left for Rome, a conquering, expansive empire where his ego would fit rather well.

▶ Rome and medicine more licentious

Galen became physician to Emperor Marcus Aurelius, but one of the first Greek doctors in Rome had been a surgeon, Archagathus, around 350 years earlier. Initial expectations were high, and high regard for Archagathus earned him citizenship, but his reputation would prove rather more for his penchant for blood than any positive outcomes for patients. Archagathus was liberal with the knife and became known quickly as 'the executioner'. In Rome, this was no mean feat. The Romans were conquerors and military strategists exacting their power, often brutally, to expand their empire.

As Rome spread to Greece its military dominance seemed unstoppable, honed in the Punic Wars against Carthage. Greece became a Roman province in 146 BC following the Battle of Corinth, and thereafter Greek physicians and intellectuals would perform their craft in Rome. Roman aestheticism came from the Greeks, aestheticism which would thereafter dim until the Renaissance. By the time Rome conquered Britain in 43 AD, Julius Caesar had been assassinated, Mark Anthony and Cleopatra had committed suicide and, shifting from republic to empire, Rome would do what it had done elsewhere: build towns and cities, bridges, aqueducts, sewage systems and villas with under-floor heating. The Romans, like ants, were unstoppable but ordered, brutal when needed, and colossal builders.

But the Romans were far less ambitious in medicine, almost dismissive of it. It might have been disapproval for Archagathus. It might have been other dispiriting false dawns; Cato the Censor (234–149 BC), for example, enthusiastically advocated cabbage for most ailments. Pliny the Elder wrote a 27-volume natural history that despised physicians. He urged capital punishment for their ignorance, while passionately describing unicorns and winged horses, before observing too closely the eruption of Vesuvius and meeting his end.

It might simply have been that preventing disease held greater sway than treatment. Sickness was invariably presumed to be the result of unhealthy living, which the Romans loathed. Rome's hospitals were principally for military purposes, with operating rooms, baths, dispensary, mortuary and herb garden. Vegetius, in a treatise on health for a Roman legion, stated only that it could avoid disease by staying out of malarial swamps and exercising regularly. Celsus wrote volumes on medicine that dwelt fleetingly on medicine and diverted lengthily into matters of food and drink.

If the Romans were less than adventuresome medically, they exceeded themselves therapeutically in one aspect of life: bathing. The Greeks bathed – *gymnasium* means '*place to get naked*' – but primarily to get clean. But the Romans were devoted to bathing with an addiction and grandeur no society had enjoyed before or has since. With their aqueducts, they had enough water to bathe on enormous scale. A *balneum* (small bathhouse) might be privately owned but open to the public. *Thermae* (larger baths) were owned by the state. The biggest, like the baths at Diocletian, could hold thousands of bathers. Fees were affordable for most free Roman men, and such was the draw of bathing that a catalogue of buildings in 354 AD documented 952 baths in Rome alone. The Romans took advantage, too, of natural springs all over Europe, including those at Bath in England.

Roman bathing was ritualistic. A bathhouse contained a series of progressively hotter rooms and pools. Most contained an *apodyterium*, a room just inside the entrance for removing clothes. The bather then gasped in the *frigidarium* (cold room), warmed in the *tepidarium* (warm room) and sweated in the *caldarium* (hot room). After these progressively perspiring immersions the bather might return to the cooler *tepidarium* for an oily massage and skin-scrub, or linger in the *laconium* (essentially a sauna).

Bathing was more than just about getting clean. Thermal waters relieved aches and pains, and overindulgence in food. Business was conducted here, and almost certainly courtship. And mostly bathing was a pastime, a way of life. Roman baths had eating places, exercise areas, libraries, perfume-sellers, beauticians and brothels. Stages held theatrical and musical performances. Bathhouses had mosaic marble floors, frescoed walls with scenes of nature, celestial domes, statuary and fountains.

As time went on mixed bathing became commonplace. Life in the baths got livelier, seemingly more lascivious. And almost certainly more liberating.

A good thing, too, for soon bathing would fall far from favour.

As would liberating behaviour.

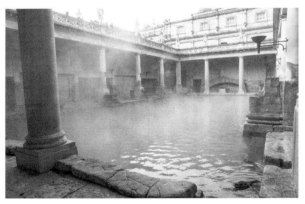

▲ Figure 3.1 Roman Baths, Bath, UK.

The Age of Darkness
and Death

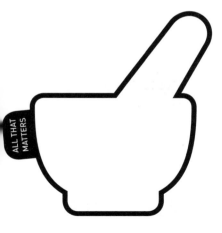

▶ The early Middle Ages

Christian and Arabian medicine

I must at once, dear reader, offer regret that this chapter sweeps through 1,000 years of history, from the fifth to fifteenth centuries: the Middle (medieval) Ages, that period spanning the end of Rome to the Renaissance. There is no room for discursive discourse, for a stray word, yet it would hardly matter if we digressed a bit (and I expect we might). It wasn't that little happened here, but little to advance medicine. These were dark days when if you weren't jolly careful you'd be burned or stoned or deadened in some other dreadful way. Medicine was heretical. Originality was a dangerous asset.

Historians debate why Rome fell. Tribes – Germanic Franks, Italian and Spanish Goths, Hun horsemen from the east and Vandals from North Africa – played their part. Constantinople, at the eastern edge of Rome's empire, was a last bastion, and its Byzantines placed a few token bricks into the enormous edifice of Graeco-Roman medicine before the early Middle Ages (500–1000) really got going. Then all of North Africa and the Middle East became Islam's empire.

Medicine passed into the hands of two polarised groups: monastic scholars of the Christian Church and Arabic scholars of pre-Islamic and Islamic worlds.

It should be said at once that 'Arabic' here refers solely to the language of physicians. Not all were native of 'Arabia'. They were from anywhere the Moslem empire extended, from Persia to Spain. Not all were Mohammedan. Many were Christian. But they began translating Greek into their language, Arabic. Galen was accepted without question. His dogmatic writing carried conviction and disarmed criticism.

The origins of Arabic medicine are often traced to the foundation of a teaching hospital at Gundeshapur (in present-day Iran) in the late fifth century. Other hospitals would appear in Baghdad, Damascus and Cairo, and Arabic medicine would enter a period of intense activity for half a millennium. Rhazes (865–925) wrote on astronomy, mathematics and medicine. His medical handbook included sections on 'slave-buying', travel advice and 'bites of venomous beasts'. Avicenna (c. 980–1037) wrote *The Canon of Medicine* (1025) with large focus on contagious diseases and *The Book of Healing* (1027), both university texts until the seventeenth century. Arabic medicine's contributions were greatest in pharmacology, famously in the formulary of Al-Kindi (800–70), and chemistry – alchemy, as it was called – but in Spain Albucasis (936–1013) stood out with his surgical encyclopaedia. Spain was home to several twelfth-century Arabic physicians, most famously Avenzoar (1094–1162), who had far-reaching influence and discovered the scabies mite, 'a very small beast, so small that he is hardly visible'. Averroes (1126–98), his pupil, wrote on poisons, including those introduced by the bites of snakes, scorpions, dogs and, 'worst of all, the bite of a fasting man'.

Against the illuminated epoch of Arabic medicine was cloistered monastic medicine. In the quiet retreat of monasteries, Greek works were transcribed by monks, and tucked away until enlightened times.

One of Christianity's first principles was healing the sick; monasteries had herb gardens growing remedies, and hospices to nurse people to health. None was more devoted to such matters than St Benedict of Nursia (480–543). Physical healing was seen as adjunctive to spiritual cure. Disease was God's will, but physicians could be agents of God, and it was permissible to seek healers. Shrines were popular. Saints, like St Blaise for throats and St Apollonia for teeth, were invoked for health. Saints Cosmos and Damian would become patrons of surgery. St Roch would preside over plague. St Hildegard of Bingen (1098–1179) is credited with many miraculous cures and treatments; for leprosy she recommended an ointment from unicorn liver, even telling readers how to catch one.

Unfortunately, Christianity was peculiarly ill at ease with bathing, indeed, with cleanliness altogether. Personal hygiene was discouraged, and Rome's obsession with bathing was a matter of unending horror. Attention to the body was considered time stolen from devotion, and being unwashed a mark of piety.

▶ The high Middle Ages

The first universities and hospitals

Arabic and Christian medicine would fuse in the Medical School of Salerno. After five centuries of comparative stagnation, medical learning formally established itself here. A seaside town south of Naples, Salerno had been a health resort since Roman times, easy to access and close to Greek-speaking lands. That it should become a meeting place for physicians and site of Europe's first organized medical school was unsurprising. Its teachers are scantily recorded, but we know that women doctors taught here, and that surgery was welcomed. In 1180 its principal exponent Rogerius (Roger Frugardi; 1140–95) wrote the surgical handbook *Practica chirurgiae* (The Practice of Surgery). Training lasted seven years.

Salerno reignited a sense of enquiry dull-wittingly absent since the Greeks, although perhaps we should demur from thinking the Middle Ages dark. In medieval art we see much humanity, with animals and babies and messy human beings. But medieval medicine operated in darkness. Diagnosis was often made in the stars. Treatment comprised bloodletting and ineffective herbs. Anatomy was taught from ancient texts. Surgery was of the meddlesome type. Learned medicine had kudos, although few practised it. The growth of Europe's towns revived demand for healers, but there was considerable overlap between village healers assimilating scraps of theory from the few academic physicians who could reason things, and academic physicians who happily incorporated unreasoned tradition into their practice.

Universities appearing by the twelfth century were allied to cathedrals. The medical school of Salerno gave place to that of Montpellier and, somewhat later, Bologna. Montpellier's most renowned teacher was Arnold of Villanova (1235–1311), who urged opening abscesses and bleeding bite wounds from mad dogs. Students came from countries afar. Famous at Bologna were physician Thaddeus Florentinus, surgeons Hugh of Lucca (1150–1257) and William of Saliceto (1210–77) and William's pupils Henri de Mondeville (c. 1260–1316) and Lanfranc of Milan (c. 1250–1306).

Other universities would appear in the picture, notably in Paris and Padua. Lanfranc would lead French surgery, and French surgery would lead surgery, Guy de Chauliac (1300–67) the most famous surgeon of later medieval times, completing his *Grand Chirurgie* in 1363. But Padua would perhaps most promote learning's renaissance; Pietro d'Abano (1257–1315) would lay its medical groundwork before dying in prison, accused of heresy.

Because care of poor and sick people (and, for Saint Francis of Assisi, animals) was incumbent upon Christians, early hospitals were ecclesiastically founded, including two London hospitals St Bartholomew's (1123) and St Thomas's (1215). Most hospitals were small, charitable institutions, more refuges than places of healing. And *leprosia* sprang up to contain the 'unclean'; by 1250 Europe had almost 20,000.

Alongside growth in learning and practice, regulation of sorts sprouted. In Paris apothecaries (early pharmacists) could only administer medicines in the presence of physicians. Valencia barbers, who also let blood, could only bleed on days physicians deemed astrologically sound. The guilds of Florence, strongly controlling trades from the twelfth to sixteenth centuries, included lawyers, wool-merchants, shoe-makers, innkeepers, sword-smiths and, collectively, physicians and pharmacists.

The medicine itself, of course, was still hopeless.

▶ The late Middle Ages

The might of the flea

Bristol was the second largest city in Britain in 1348 and the principal port for the West Country. Conditions were as in any medieval town: chamber pots were emptied from windows, water was drawn from the river and pigs lived in houses.

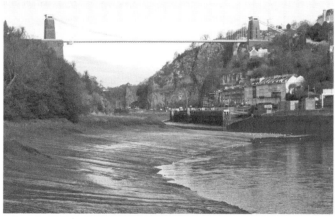

▲ Figure 4.1 River Avon, Clifton, Bristol: entry point of plague to Britain, 1348.

Rumours of a terrible plague sweeping across Europe had rumbled for some time. Perhaps predictably Bristol was the first major town in Britain to let it in. The Black Death would arrive and flourish here.

It was not until the end of the nineteenth century that *Yersinia pestis* was identified as the cause of plague, transmitted by the bites of fleas carried by black rats. Bubonic plague provoked swellings or buboes as big as eggs in the neck, groin or armpit, while pneumonic plague overwhelmed the respiratory system. Within days plague killed most it infected.

By 1300 plague was rampaging through Asia before sweeping westwards to the Middle East, North Africa and Europe. Leprosy was no longer the scourge to fear. By 1347 plague was in Italy and France. In the summer of 1348 it reached England. By 1349 a third to a half of Europe's people were dead. In Bristol the grass grew long in silent streets.

Pessimism prevailed, and all enquiring minds came to the wrong conclusion. Plague was mostly attributed to something bad in the air: doors and windows were shut and sealed, aromas burned and sponges soaked in vinegar for those who went out. Many agreed that bathing opened pores, allowing deadly vapours into the body, and plugged their pores with dirt. Some believed that water was polluted with spiders or lizards, or the flesh of snakes. Scapegoats were sought in lepers, the poor, the wealthy, the clergy and, most popularly, Jews. Commonly plague was seen as chastisement from God. Avoidance of unchaste living became an obsession. Self-flagellation was rife. Most flagellants were men, who spurned the company of women and sought to purge themselves of sin. Sometimes it was performed en masse, notably in Italy.

The Black Death brought unrest. France and England experienced uprisings and a century of undulating conflict. Days were as dark as they could be. Everybody had been touched by death, disease or despair.

The Ages of 'Early Modern' Medicine

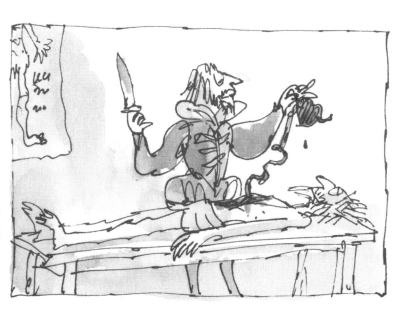

"Early Modern"

5

The Age of Anatomy

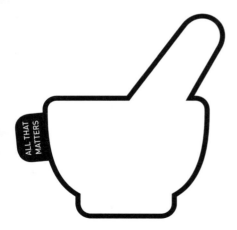

ALL THAT MATTERS

► Exploration of the natural world

The Dark Ages ended with a dawn in exploration. In 1492 Christopher Columbus (1451–1506) reached Hispaniola, today's Dominican Republic and Haiti, but Old and New World engagement would bring biological catastrophe.

The first New World epidemic was probably a type of swine influenza harboured by pigs aboard Columbus's vessels. Smallpox reached the Caribbean in 1518, killing almost half of Hispaniola's population. When Cortés encountered the Aztecs a year later, its emperor believed him a manifestation of their god Quetzalcoatl and offered little resistance. Half of Tenochtitlán's 300,000 Aztecs were dead within months, attacked and diseased (though doubtless the Spaniards were aided by those tired of the Aztecs' insatiable desire for human sacrifice). The Incas incurred a similar fate ten years later. Typhus, measles and more influenza followed. Parts of America saw peoples almost disappear, driving Spanish and Portuguese conquerors to import slaves from Africa, and in the process malaria and yellow fever.

Other than gold, Columbus's voyage arguably delivered a more deadly consignment from the New World: syphilis. The first European outbreak was in 1495 at the siege of Naples, many Spanish soldiers recently having returned from the New World. Genital ulcers and rash progressed, with unnerving unpredictability, to abscesses, dissolving bones and face. The new disease spread like wildfire, slaying many and committing others to ultimate 'madness' and death.

One thing Europeans found solace in contemplating, in happy reprieve from plagues and wars, was nature. It was with no small excitement that new species appeared from voyages. By 1565, Spanish physician Nicolás Monardes (1493–1588) was claiming, in *Two Books on All the Things*

Found in our West Indies, that America's plants were worth more than its gold. Monardes had published previous works endorsing Classical medicine, and the less expansive *De Rosa et partibus eius* about roses and citrus fruits. But his twin-volume account of West Indian naturalia would find him at his most effusive, for that naturalia included, as well as the contestably forgettable sassafras and sarsaparilla, the more incontestably captivating coca and tobacco. Monardes took to his grave the conviction that tobacco would be an infallible cure for everything, a notion that probably spurred his most notable work, the three-part *Historia medicinal de las cosas que se traen de nuestras Indias Occidentales* (Medical Study of the Products Imported from our West Indian Possessions). It would be translated widely into Latin and English as *Joyfull News out of the New Found World*, as those in the Old World began to appreciate tobacco as much as Monardes. And then there was guaiac wood, which held promise for syphilis.

Novel to Europeans, the 'great pox' (distinguished from smallpox) was known as the 'French disease' to the Spanish and 'the Spanish' disease to the French. Few if any considered it infective, or to have emerged from the exploits of exploration. Some attributed it to planetary alignment, while others blamed lepers and a few, perhaps more accurately albeit missing the point, prostitutes.

▶ Renaissance medicine

Exploration would be one torch out of centuries of darkness. The Renaissance would be the other. Europe's 'rebirth' was not just a revival in Classical Greek and Roman culture. It brought freedom of thought and serious enquiry. It started in late medieval Italy, notably Florence. Giotto's frescoes in Padua (1305) were among the first Renaissance paintings. 1408 brought Donatello's statue *David*, 1486 Botticelli's *Birth of Venus*. In the early 1500s Michelangelo painted the Sistine Chapel and Leonardo da Vinci the *Mona Lisa*.

Medicine limped behind art like a ragged dog. It was practised by physicians, barbers and village herbalists, loosely integrated, and still steeped in magic. Practitioners conducted consultations in early 'surgeries', making improbable diagnoses and issuing incorrect prescriptions. Apothecaries formulated and dispensed drugs. Some gave medical advice. Some performed surgery. Many sold tobacco. Women developed 'expertise' in 'homely' matters like childbirth.

In these times lived a strange man whose influence upon medicine's progress is difficult to assess. The prevailing opinion of Swiss physician Philippus Aureolus Theophrastus Bombastus von Hohenheim (1493–1541), who preferred to be known as Paracelsus – 'beyond (by which von Hohenheim meant 'better than') Roman authority Celsus' – was that he was a disreputable braggart, while more kindly descriptions spoke of his unsound mind. He travelled far and wide, even to Cornish tin mines (sparsely populous, which might tell us something about his receptivity, doubtless not helped in Italy by his insistence on lecturing in German), and always carried a sword. All body processes, he asserted, were driven by chemistry, and specifically just three chemicals: mercury, sulfur and salt. All disease, he decided, was a result of their maladjustment: basically there were three diseases and three remedies. More helpfully, Paracelsus preached on astronomy (not the prevailing astrology), and in alchemy he envisaged medicine's philosopher's stone.

Alongside Paracelsus, other physicians merit mention. Gerolamo Cardan (1501–76) has no lasting legacy but was perhaps the most admired sixteenth-century physician. Thomas Linacre (1460–1524), concerned that medicine in England was endangered by the empiricism of illiterate practitioners, obtained letters of patent for a body of physicians that would become (1551) the Royal College of Physicians of London. Girolamo Fracastoro (Fracastorius; 1478–1553) gave syphilis its name in a poem, was first to recognize typhus and developed a flair for epidemiological thinking, demonstrated in *De Contagione* (On Contagion). Long before knowledge of microbes, he presumed the existence of imperceptible particles or 'seminaria', seeds of disease, which 'multiply rapidly and propagate their like.'

In Naples, Bologna, Florence, Venice, Rome and elsewhere hospitals were helping the poor, old and sick. Some were former plague hospitals. Some were new. Most were charitable. Europe was largely liberated from leprosy. Plague had completed its cull. Now there was space for the chronic 'incurables', and the insane, often due to syphilis. In the fifteenth century, Florence had had over 30 hospitals. By 1500, though scant outside major cities, there were over 500 in England. England's hospital flame might have burned as brightly as Italy's, but the Henrician Reformation and Protestantism ('protest' against Rome) from 1536 dissolved monasteries and closed most foundations (church-administered), and so it flickered and fizzled. In Catholic countries – Italy, Spain and France – hospitals multiplied. The Hôtel-Dieu in Paris became the world's largest, run by religious orders, and throughout France 'hospitals' would sprout everywhere in the 1600s, some for the sick, many shelters for orphans, vagabonds and prostitutes. In 1588 England defeated the Spanish Armada. Drake would later circumnavigate the world. But hospitals were like unwanted puppies. A smattering re-emerged on a secular basis, including St Bartholomew's and St Thomas's, and Bethlam (Bedlam), Britain's only lunatic asylum. But outside London there would be no hospitals (although puppies in abundance) in Britain until after 1700.

▶ Vesalius's anatomy

If you were really searching for a lighthouse in medicine's darkness, you would need to do so in Italy. The first documented human dissection took place in Bologna in

1315 by Mondino de' Luzzi (1270–1326). *Mondino's Anatomy* became the standard text to be read out in class, dealing with the body in order of most to least perishable, abdominal contents handled first. Mondino perpetuated Galen's animal dissection errors, but unleashed a wave of anatomical teaching across Italy. Anatomy theatres were built. Public dissections were staged by learned professors. Winter was preferred, to delay putrefaction, the corpses of executed criminals often used as final acts of punishment. Early illustrations show a robed professor in an elevated chair overseeing dissection, reciting a text, probably Mondino's, while a surgeon slits the cadaver and an assistant indicates features with a pointer. Anatomy was both education and spectacle. Dissection proved so popular that artists, too, took it up. By 1500 da Vinci and Michelangelo were performing dissections and illustrating what they found.

In 1543 *De Fabrica Corporis Humani* (On the Construction of the Human Body) caused quite a stir. Its author, Flemish anatomist Andreas Vesalius (1514–64), studied in Paris, Louvain and Padua, and at once became professor of anatomy and surgery (in that day anatomists were surgeons). Driven and confident, enquiring and exacting, Vesalius attacked orthodoxy, particularly animal dissections; Vesalius's teacher Jacques Dubois had taught from dog limbs and been so adherent to Galen that, if he found any structure not conforming to Galen's description, he alleged that the human body had changed since Galen's time.

Vesalius promoted a new sense of observation in human dissections that led to accurate descriptions of organs and systems. What made *De Fabrica* so novel, however, were its exquisite illustrations. Vesalius recognized that, to really edify a subject, physician and artist must collaborate. Vesalius's collaborator was German-born Italian painter Jan van Calcar who produced the eloquent woodcuts for *De Fabrica*.

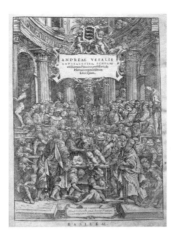

▲ Figure 5.1 Vesalius teaching anatomy. Title page of De Fabrica Corporis Humani. 1543. British Library.

Vesalius's work inspired the next generation. His successor at Padua, Realdo Colombo (1516–59), described the pulmonary circulation in *De re Anatomica* (On Anatomy; 1559). Gabriele Falloppio (1523–63), successor after Colombo's brief interregnum, was equally anatomically adept, not least when it came to female genitalia. He named the vagina, described the clitoris and delineated the tubes connecting ovaries to uterus to which he gave his name. He went to his grave, however, without notion of the functions of anything he found.

And so the sixteenth century closed with an explosion of knowledge. Bartolomeo Eustachio discovered the Eustachian tube, Girolamo Fabrizio (Fallopio's successor) valves in veins, Gaspare Aselli lacteal vessels. The human body's design became intricately known. But what the parts did remained elusive. Not least the fallopian tubes. And not least, for that matter, the clitoris. It caused fierce debate. Vesalius argued against the existence of a clitoris in normal women. Colombo claimed to have discovered it, though had not named it. Falloppio disputed this, claiming its discovery, though not its function.

6

The Age of Blood, Bodies and Battles

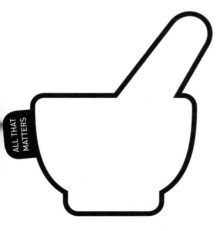

▶ Harvey and a new dawn

It was easier to deduce anatomy than grasp the functions of things. It would fall to an Englishman, William Harvey (1578–1657), to demonstrate that blood circulated, transforming anatomy into an enquiry about process.

Galen had said that blood was created in the liver, dispersing through veins like water irrigating fields to nourish the body. A separate arterial system carried blood and air from the heart, distributing life to the peripheries. Like bellows, the lungs fanned and cooled arterial blood. The portion of venous blood joining the right side of the heart divided into two, some nourishing the lungs, the remainder passing through septal pores to the left side of the heart to mix with air and pass to the peripheries and out through pores in the skin.

Galen's theory had obvious flaws. One was that the heart's septum was solid. For blood to pass from right to left it would have to circumnavigate the heart. Spanish physician Michael Servetus (1509–53) had, in 1553, proposed a 'pulmonary' circulation (for which he was burned for heresy) before Colombo. Another flaw in Galen's theory was that it required too much blood to make sense.

Harvey observed the hearts of animal after animal: eel, snail, shrimp, chick-before-hatching, pigeon and, most usefully, frog (the slow heartbeat, unlike in warm-blooded animals, facilitated observation). He noted that the volume of blood expelled from the heart of any animal in one hour far exceeded the volume in that animal. Hundreds of gallons of blood could not conceivably be absorbed by the body and remade in the liver. 'It is absolutely necessary to conclude that the blood in the animal body is impelled in a circle, and is in a state of ceaseless motion,' he concluded.

Harvey graduated from Cambridge in 1597, studied under Fabrizio in Padua, became Fellow of the Royal College of

Physicians and was thence appointed to St Bartholomew's Hospital (attending the poor once a week in its hall with fireplace stoked by Windsor forest wood). By 1603 Harvey could say that 'the movement of the blood occurs constantly in a circular manner and is the result of the beating of the heart'. In 1616 he lectured on pulmonary transit, the simultaneous contractions of the heart's ventricles and the shock waves pulsing through arteries. The findings were published in *Exercitatio Anatomica de Motu Cordis et Sanguinis* (An Anatomical Disquisition on the Motion of the Heart and Blood; 1628).

One thing Harvey could not demonstrate were capillaries, the tiny peripheral conduits between arteries and veins. The microscope was developing but Harvey's surrogate method of demonstrating flow at microscopic level was achieved with a series of ligatures: those tight enough to occlude arterial and venous flow did not result in swelling of the arm; those merely occluding veins, more superficial than arteries, allowed blood to flow into the arm but not out, resulting in swelling. And a series of finger pressure demonstrations showed that valves in veins always directed blood towards the heart.

Harvey's clinical practice suffered. The world was on the cusp of a scientific revolution. But Harvey, seen as unorthodox, was just a little ahead of his time.

▶ Plagues, fires and witches

Early in September 1665 George Viccars, a tailor, opened a consignment of cloth in his cottage in the Derbyshire village of Eyam. It was damp so he hung it out in front of his fire to dry.

Within days he was dead.

By the end of September, five more villagers succumbed similarly, and by the end of October the toll was 23.

Viccars' package had come from London, where bubonic plague had raged for months, the cloth containing fleas in which plague's bacterium harboured. Many villagers, stricken by panic, prepared to leave, but fearing spread of plague Eyam's two clergymen urged villagers to remain until the scourge was over. The village sealed itself off from the world. Piled stones marked its boundaries. Supplies of food from outside were left at the stones, remunerated by coins placed in jars of disinfecting vinegar. By the following summer, two-thirds of Eyam's population was dead, its cemetery full, and people were buried in fields.

Plague had provoked quarantine, a word derived from the number 40 (in Venetian, *quaranta*), the number of days suspected sick people were isolated.

In the 'early modern' world devastating diseases appeared, and mysteriously disappeared. Plague would reappear for its last disconcerting bout in Europe in 1720, in Asia a century later. The English sweating sickness, a disease about which we know little, arrived in epidemics through the early 1500s, with a less uniformly fatal outcome than plague but, by all accounts, substantial sweats. It originally broke out among the soldiers of Henry VII in 1485, about to inaugurate the Tudor dynasty, when 'not one in a hundred escaped'. Epidemics recurred in the summers of 1508, 1517, 1528 and 1551. It has never come back, but was followed shortly by another fever – 'the great death' – which 'killed an exceeding great number of all sorts of men, but especially gentlemen and men of great wealth', according to one early source. All manner of measures were tried by those with diseases to alleviate themselves. Writer Bernard Bluet d'Arbères starved himself to death in the Parisian plague of 1606. In the English 'plague year' (1665) people threw themselves from windows, plunged into the river or shot themselves. London's Great Fire of 1666 doubtless killed many fleas.

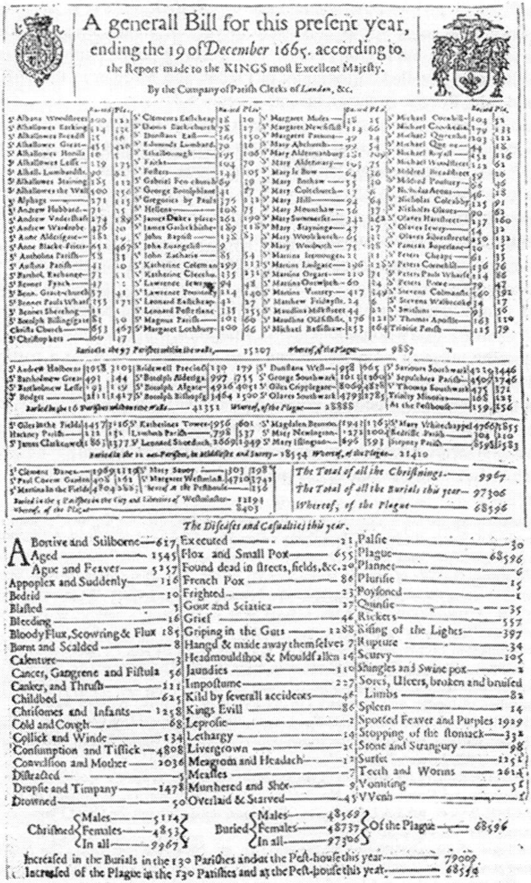

A generall Bill for this present year, ending the 19 of *December* 1665. according to the Report made to the KINGS most Excellent Majesty.

By the Company of Parish Clerks of *London*, &c.

Buried in the 97 Parishes within the walls, —— 15207 *Whereof, of the Plague* —— 9887

Buried in the 16 Parishes without the Walls —— 41351 *Whereof, of the Plague* —— 28888

Buried in the 12 out-Parishes, in Middlesex and Surrey – 18554 *Whereof, of the Plague* – 21420

Buried in the 5 Parishes in the City and Liberties of Westminster – 12194
Whereof, of the Plague —— 8403

The Total of all the Christnings. —— 9967
The Total of all the Burials this year — 97306
Whereof, of the Plague —— 68596

The Diseases and Casualties this year.

ABortive and Stilborne	617	Executed	21	Palsie	30
Aged	1545	Flox and Small Pox	655	Plague	68596
Ague and Feaver	5257	Found dead in streets, fields, &c.	20	Plannet	6
Appoplex and Suddenly	116	French Pox	86	Plurisie	15
Bedrid	10	Frighted	23	Poysoned	1
Blasted	5	Gout and Sciatica	27	Quinsie	35
Bleeding	16	Grief	46	Rickets	557
Bloody Flux, Scowring & Flux	185	Griping in the Guts	1288	Rising of the Lights	397
Burnt and Scalded	8	Hangd & made away themselves	7	Rupture	34
Calenture	3	Headmouldshot & Mouldfallen	14	Scurvy	105
Cancer, Gangrene and Fistula	56	Jaundies	110	Shingles and Swine pox	2
Canker, and Thrush	111	Impostume	227	Sores, Ulcers, broken and bruised Limbs	82
Childbed	625	Kild by severall accidents	46	Spleen	14
Chrisomes and Infants	1258	Kings Evill	86	Spotted Feaver and Purples	1929
Cold and Cough	68	Leprosie	2	Stopping of the stomack	332
Collick and Winde	134	Lethargy	14	Stone and Strangury	98
Consumption and Tissick	4808	Livergrown	20	Surfet	1251
Convulsion and Mother	2036	Meagrom and Headach	12	Teeth and Worms	2614
Distracted	5	Measles	7	Vomiting	51
Dropsie and Timpany	1478	Murthered and Shot	9	VVenn	1
Drowned	50	Overlaid & Starved	45		

Christned { Males —— 5114, Females —— 4853, In all —— 9967 }
Buried { Males —— 48569, Females —— 48737, In all —— 97306 } Of the Plague —— 68596

Increased in the Burials in the 130 Parishes and at the Pest-house this year —— 79009
Increased of the Plague in the 130 Parishes and at the Pest-house this year —— 68590

▲ Figure 6.1 Bill of mortality, London 1665. Wellcome Library. This City of London's death roll makes intriguing inspection. Most deaths, as might be expected, were from plague, but others included the unenviable *murthered and shot* and *stone and strangury*, the unfortunate *frighted*, the unexciting *bedrid*, and the unexpectedly unnerving *griping in the guts*.

In the 1570s Bath and Buxton were popular spas in England, bathhouses having enjoyed a modest resurgence. It was short-lived. Many people remained convinced of the licentiousness of time spent washing instead of praying. Others felt the communal pleasure of water risky. Although people recognized that syphilis was spread by sexual contact, they associated it mostly with bathhouses. Firstly, prostitutes were banned from bathhouses, and then everyone was banned from bathhouses, which closed all across Europe (while sexual activity continued widely). Without any notion of micro-organisms – many of which thrive in water (consider the cholera and polio epidemics yet to come) – water, and washing in particular, came to be regarded with scepticism for all the wrong reasons. In particular, water was thought to transmit disease through the skin's pores, and so protective layers of dirt were regarded comfortingly. Most people stopped washing altogether, not that they had been doing so with enthusiasm. Elizabeth I bathed once a month, as did Marie Antionette. Louis XIV succeeded most of his life without a bath. And scientist Robert Hooke appears to have enjoyed bathing up to his ankles but very little else. Bathing fingers, and occasionally toes, seems to have been the most that most would allow themselves. Hooke, oddly enough, would be among the first to witness the microbiological world through the microscope, a hundred years after Fracastorius had mooted the idea of germs and two hundred years before anyone took any notice.

In short, infections were everywhere. And people stank everywhere. But the prevailing view was that where everybody stank, nobody stank.

Instead of germs, witchery often seemed to be behind the coming of disease. In Salem, Massachusetts in 1692, 13 women and six men were executed for witchcraft after people became delirious and crazed, probably due to poisoning by the rye-grain fungus, ergot. People ingesting the fungus and developing ergotism often died, having previously developed a cough like a dog's bark (thought to be the origin of the expression 'barking mad').

Since ideas about witchcraft and heresy remained strong in parts of Europe, notably England well into the 1600s, medicine was greatly retarded, but notable physicians of the age included Thomas Sydenham from Dorset (who dismissed textbooks, advised students to read Don Quixote and encouraged them to the bedside) and Thomas Dover (ship surgeon and rescuer of Alexander Selkirk, the inspiration for Robinson Crusoe).

▶ Surgery so far

Sir Kenelm Digby (1603–65), aside from sporting a rather eccentric name, had rather eccentric ideas. Born at Gayhurst, Buckinghamshire, his father was of 'gentry stock' and was executed in 1606 for a part in the Gunpowder Plot. Digby spent his early adulthood in Europe, where Marie de' Medici, he asserted, 'fell madly in love with him'. In 1625 he married not Medici but Venetia Stanley, whose wooing he described exactingly in memoirs. His political views were whatever his future demanded. A staunch Roman Catholic, eager to become a member of Charles I's Privy Council, he switched to Anglicanism, a requisite for government office. In 1628 he became an adventurer, stealing foreign ships, before returning to England to administer naval affairs. Venetia died suddenly in 1633, and stricken with grief (and, for reasons of which history tells us little, object of enough suspicion for the Crown to order an autopsy, rare at the time), Digby secluded himself in scientific experimentation. He spent time in exile in Paris but, following an incident in which he killed a French nobleman in a duel, returned to England and at the Restoration found himself in favour with the new regime. He was regarded as eccentric, partly because of his effusive personality, and partly because of his interests in matters scientific. His life straddled a time when scientific enquiry had not settled down in any disciplined way. He delved in astrology and alchemy, and notably promoted a wound salve. To heal rapier wounds, this mixture of earthworms, pig's brain and powdered embalmed corpses, mixed with nitric oxide (and, seemingly, anything one fancied) was daubed not on the wound but on the weapon and said to work by 'sympathetic' magic. His book on the salve went through 29 editions, and its popularity demonstrated surgery's shortcomings. Perhaps Digby's most useful literary legacy was *The Closet of the Eminently Learned Sir Kenelme Digbie Knight Opened*, a cookbook, written posthumously by a servant. He also, apparently, devised the wine bottle.

Before the introduction of anaesthesia, surgery's scope would be woefully restrained. Wound management was ever-controversial, though perhaps no argument would, through history's retrospect, seem less persuasive than Digby's salve. The removal of pus had been advocated by Henri de Mondeville and Guy de Chauliac in the late Middle Ages, de Chaliac's *Grand Chirurgie* the prime surgical text for two centuries.

Battlefields proved the most potent schools of surgery. Gunpowder, invented in the late Middle Ages, complicated the character of wounds. Gangrenous limbs eventually needed amputation, but before the sixteenth century blood loss made any amputation above the knee universally fatal.

Civilian surgery, meanwhile, was undertaken by barbers, as well as quacks purporting specific skills, and oculists who did an array of things with cataracts to render vision worse.

Proverbially, good surgery required an eagle's eye, a lion's heart and a woman's hand, though most patients would have fared better without the lion's heart. But by the sixteenth century, surgery was at least becoming more organized. In 1540 the Fellowship of Surgeons – then a distinct profession – merged with the Company of Barbers to form the Company of Barber-Surgeons, which would exist for 200 years. Ambroise Paré (1510–90) had Vesalius's teachings translated into French and, a barber-surgeon himself with skills honed on battlefields, devised the ligature to stem bleeding at amputations and an ointment of egg yolk, rose oil and turpentine for open wounds which proved more effective (and less excruciating) than hot oil. Paré and Vesalius would meet in 1559 at Henry II of France's deathbed. The king had been fatally wounded in the head by a lance, the most eminent surgeon and most flamboyant anatomist of the day summoned to his aid. Queen Catherine, desperate to determine the nature of the injury and find a cure for her husband, 'had four criminals beheaded and broken truncheons thrust into the eyes of the corpses at the appropriate angle of penetration'.

Paré relayed his wound experiences in *Method of Treating Wounds* (1545). Then, in 1563, Thomas Gale's *Treatise of Wounds with Gonneshot* appeared. Later, John Woodall's *The Surgeon's Mate* (1617) and Richard Wiseman's *Several Chirurgical Treatises* (1676) shared experiences from naval battles and the English Civil War, revealing the grim reality of amputation on bloody battlefields and storm-whipped seas.

7

The Age of Science

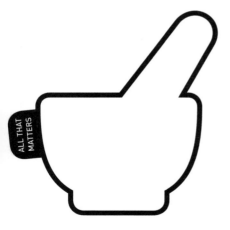

▶ The scientific revolution

Harvey's work was viewed suspiciously for some time, notably in Paris where French physicians remained loyal to Galen or, perhaps more likely, reluctant to espouse the assertions of an Englishman.

But Harvey's ideas touched a batch of new investigators in England, not least anatomist Thomas Willis (1621–73) who, as well as fathering nine children, studied the nervous system in detail and gave us both the word 'neurologie' and his pupil Richard Lower (1631–91) from Cornwall's Camel Valley. The question left by Harvey was why blood circulated. The answer was found, step by step, by a quartet of young Oxford scientists fuelling the new field of physiology. Lower was convinced that air in the lungs turned dark venous blood into bright arterial blood. Another Cornishman, John Mayow (1641–79), would describe the mechanics of breathing and postulate that blood carried something vital from air. Robert Boyle (1626–91), best known for laws on gas volumes and pressures, had shown that mice and small birds fared better in air (in which they were unperturbed) than in vacuums (in which they died). While Boyle's assistant, Robert Hooke (1635–1703), observing Boyle's experiments, concluded that air must be important, and claimed the idea for himself.

A scientific revolution had been ignited, a revolution seeded in the previous century with Vesalius's anatomy, and works like Falloppio's *Anatomical Observations* and Conrad Gesner's *Histories of Animals*. Now René Descartes's rationalist philosophy gave science impetus, as did Galileo's cosmologies, Francis Bacon's *Novum Organum* outlining scientific method, and, pivotally, Harvey's work. The formative seal of the revolution was the founding in 1660 of The Royal Society ('for Improving Natural Knowledge'). Its founding members included Willis, Lower, Mayow, Boyle, Hooke and Kenelm Digby (whom we last met preparing an improbable

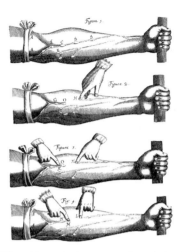

▲ Figure 7.1 William Harvey's demonstration of circulation.

wound salve, now engaged in correspondence about Pythagorean triangles and his *Discourse Concerning the Vegetation of Plants* asserting that air seemed important for plants). The Society met weekly to discuss the 'new science' and conduct experiments. Its Curator of Experiments was Hooke. From a poor background, through wits and curiosity Hooke became a skilled scientist, and after science's success in transfusing blood from one dog into another (the recipient seemed more energetic) but some seriously unwelcome outcomes when blood was exchanged between humans (and on one occasion from a lamb), Hooke's task at the Royal Society's meetings was to entertain and educate with less deadly experiments.

In the early 1600s the concept of the 'body machine' arose. Physics was developing apace, with figures like Boyle and then Newton (though Newton's reputation would need time to ferment, in 1686 the Royal Society publishing Francis Willughby's *History of Fishes* rather than Newton's theories). Hydrostatic pressures conveniently explained the movement of fluids in the body's vessels, and Giovanni Borelli (1608–79) was one of numerous scientists arguing that mechanics was the key to life. In *De Motu Animalium* (On Animal Motion; 1680) he recorded his observations on muscle contraction, breathing, bird flight and swimming fish. Everything in life, he affirmed, was a mechanical process, an idea seemingly beloved of many Italians. Gjuro Baglivi (1668–1707), Rome's professor of anatomy, proclaimed: 'A human body, as to its natural actions, is truly nothing else but a complex of chymico-mechanical motions, depending on such principles as are purely mathematical.' The view was opposed by Paracelsus's follower Johannnes Baptista van Helmont (1597–1644), who held chemistry as life's key. The Royal Society would be pivotal in putting these polarized ideas into science's roomy crucible, in which other things such as cells were coming into the mix.

▶ Cells!

The first person to identify a cell was Hooke. He described the little chambers in plants as 'cells', for they resembled to him monks' cells, and calculated that a one-inch square of cork would contain 1,259,712,000 cells, a number almost incalculably large even to respecting scientists of the day. Microscopes had been around since the late 1500s, but now – in no small part because of modifications devised by Hooke – offered magnifications of 30 times. All of a sudden, physical and chemical concepts of the workings of the body were enhanced by something preposterously novel and exciting: a microscopic world underlying the macroscopic one, hitherto the only one known. Hooke was protective of his findings, due in no small part to a suspicious mind. In 1683, when scientists were musing over celestial motion, a prize was offered to whomever could solve the puzzle of why planets were inclined to orbit in an ellipse. Hooke claimed to have solved the puzzle, but declined to share it, arguing altruistically that the others should not be denied the edifying experience of solving it for themselves. Hooke was fond of being first in things, although his book *Microphagia: Some Physiological Descriptions of Miniature Bodies Made by Magnifying Glasses* (1665) almost two decades earlier was unquestionably groundbreaking.

Equally unquestionable was the rivalry between Hooke and others with access to a microscope. Marcello Malpighi (1628–94) of Bologna was able to demonstrate the structure of the lungs and see the capillaries linking arteries and veins that had eluded Harvey. He shed light on the liver, spleen, skin and brain, as well as inexhaustible arrays of pond-life. Jan Swammerdam (1637–80), with no training in anything, made the largest, most beautiful illustrations of insects, not least dragonflies, and their organs. But what perturbed Hooke most was when the Royal Society began receiving drawings from a linen draper in the Netherlands, Anton van Leeuwenhoek (1632–1723), with evident access to a resolution greater than anything Hooke had devised. Van Leeuwenhoek's drawings are all the more surprising because his device was little more than a magnifying glass, far less a microscope, but over a period of 50 years he would report regularly to the Royal Society, submitting drawings of unparalleled detail. All sorts of things were unearthed in this enchanting miniature world – mould, algae, insect parts, coffee bean interiors, red blood cells, muscle fibres, tooth plaque, faeces and spermatozoa – and presented (the latter with fearful apology if considered scandalous or repugnant) to the Royal Society.

▶ Scientific 'continuation'

Physiologists and pathologists

It had been long noted by some living on coasts that crabs and lobsters, upon losing a claw or scale, produced another in its stead. The notion was widely disbelieved but Parisian René

Réaumur (1683–1757) ended the dispute in 1712 by removing a claw and observing its regrowth. Réaumur's papers covered many aspects of science: his first, in 1708, on geometry; his last, in 1756, on birds' nests; in between he proved that the strength of a rope is more than the sum of the strengths of its strands, reported on auriferous rivers and wrote about spiders.

The Enlightenment was a period of intellectual consolidation in Europe, originating towards the end of the seventeenth century and continuing throughout the eighteenth. Europe's population was growing. Thinking was diversifying. Science was making its mark in physics and the natural sciences.

Swedish physician and naturalist Carl Linnaeus (1707–78) developed a classification of organisms. Doubtless the most ingenious classification ever devised, its nomenclature exhibited a certain preoccupation. Parts of a clam he named 'vulva', 'labia', 'pubes', 'anus', and 'hymen'; his conchology (pertaining to the shells of molluscs) consistently contained 'buttocks'. He named a plant genus *Clitoria*. *Fornicata* appeared with remarkable regularity, while *Clitoria* and *Vulva* recurrently reappeared. His system is now so established we give it little thought, but before Linnaeus there was no scientific classification ('taxonomy'). Animals were categorized as large or small, fierce or tame, important or of no consequence, or with respect to traits like handsomeness and countenance. Even Linnaeus accommodated 'mythical beasts' (science being still in its infancy, dragons were still thought to reside reclusively in the Alps). Linnaeus's first edition of *Systema Naturae* (1735) occupied 14 pages, his twelfth (1760), the last of his lifetime, 2,300. Linnaeus divided the animal world into six categories: mammals; birds; reptiles; fish; insects; and, for everything that didn't fit, worms. Anything that didn't fit could not endure being catalogued as a worm, and the system would need some adjusting, but the broad system of kingdom, phylum, class, order, family, genus and species that developed, has endured (and amply accommodates worms).

Latin taxonomy would soon embrace human anatomy. Anatomy built on Vesalius's mergence of science and art, with eloquent atlases of the human body produced. And medical parties quarrelled vigorously. Herman Boerhaave (1668–1738), professor at Leiden, saw the body as a series of perfectly balanced systems in which pressures and flows in liquids were crucial. Smooth fluid mechanics were felt integral to health, while blockages created disease. But the presence of a soul also seemed indisputable.

The 'secret of life' became far from idle speculation. Réaumur's experiment would form part of the debate as to whether a living organism was more than a mere machine. That it was something more was cemented by Swiss naturalist Abraham Trembley (1710–84) who found that dividing freshwater polyps (hydra) created completely new individuals. Trembley, whose laboratory contained hundreds of jars of animals, is considered by some to have pioneered biology. His hydra findings, however, had been presaged, perhaps predictably, by Van Leeuwenhoek. Van Leeuwenhoek, insatiably curious, had already described the process of hydra budding in a 1702–3 volume of *Philosophical Transactions of the Royal Society*.

Experimentation was everywhere in this new age. Albrecht von Haller's *Elementa Physiologiae Corporis Humani* (Elements of the Physiology of the Human Body; 1759–66) pronounced that muscles contracted in response to stimuli and that nerves responded to pain, the concepts of irritability and sensibility laying the foundations of neurophysiology.

Physiology (then called 'animal economy') – the study of how the body functioned – was of integral interest in Edinburgh's new medical school. Inspired by Haller, Edinburgh's professor of medicine, William Cullen (1710–90), proposed that nervous energy fuelled life itself and that all disease arose from a nervous system gone awry. John Brown (1735–88), Cullen's successor, reduced the argument to abject simplicity: a state of health or sickness was a product of the degree of excitability of the body, sthenic states being rather more excitable, asthenic states rather less so. What made Brown's argument especially appealing was that either state could be cured with the correct balance of alcohol and opium.

Medicine, and particularly physiology, was aided by all emerging sciences of the period. Gas chemistry revealed that different air entered and exited the lungs. Luigi Galvani (1737–98) amused himself and then the world with experiments on dead frogs' legs, demonstrating movement if stimulated with electrical impulses, providing argument for an electrical life-force as well as inspiration for Mary Shelley's *Frankenstein*.

Physiology (the normal workings of the body) would lead to interest in pathophysiology (its abnormal workings) and pathology (disease demonstrable within organs). That, after all, might aid physicians dealing with disease. The transition was given impetus by Giovanni Morgagni (1682–1771), anatomy professor at Padua. His *De Sedibus et Causis Morborum* (On the Sites and Causes of Disease; 1761) drew on hundreds of autopsies and case histories that would start relating disease found in organs to clinical manifestations, both symptoms (the experiences of the patient) and signs (the findings of the doctor through examination). His most notable finding was arteriosclerosis (hardening of the arteries).

Morgagni's work was transformational, and foundational for those who followed. Matthew Baillie's *The Morbid Anatomy of Some of the Most Important Parts of the Human Body* (1793) included descriptions of emphysema of the lungs, alcoholic cirrhosis of the liver and rheumatic heart disease. And Marie François Xavier Bichat (1771–1802) inoculated the idea that disease arose from the microscopic tissues that made up organs, not organs per se, and gave histopathology its enduring relevance.

8

The Age of Expansion in Medicine and Surgery

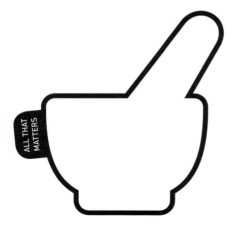

▶ Physicians and quacks

Physicians (often physiologists themselves) flourished in the 1700s from the emerging physiological science. Schools at Edinburgh, Vienna and Leiden blossomed with big names and big ideas, too many to mention. Alexander Monro (primus) founded Edinburgh's medical school in 1726. William Heberden (1710–1801), physician to George III, described angina. William Withering (1741–99) described digitalis in *Account of the Foxglove*. James Currie (1756–1805) introduced thermometry, on typhoid patients, while the Reverend Stephen Hales (1677–1761), a versatile English clergyman, had been first to measure blood pressure by inserting a glass tube into the artery of a horse. Edinburgh's John Fothergill (1712–80) wrote *An Account of the Sore Throat, History and Use of Coffee and Weather and Disease* and discovered that artificial respiration could 'revive the dead'. At the same time in Vienna Leopold Auenbrugger (1722–1809) discovered the usefulness of chest percussion in detecting signs in the living.

John Morgan (1735–89), with William Shippen (1712–1801), founded Pennsylvania's school of medicine (and thus American medical education) in 1765 in his native Philadelphia after training in Edinburgh. The American Revolution would further organize medicine in the United States.

As science unfolded, so came new cures. Calomel was popular, and combined with wine, laxative salts, opium and castor oil said to cleanse the body of foul liquids. It provoked unrestrained salivation and bowel evacuation. Unsurprisingly, people feared and scorned doctors, whose 'cures' often killed.

And so the eighteenth century provided a perfect canvas for the art of quackery (in the Middle Ages, 'quacksalver' denoted someone noisily 'quacking' and selling 'salves' on the street) when all manner of cures were touted for all manner of ills. Charlatans were often small time, but Joshua Ward's 'drops' and 'pills' brought him handsome reward. Unqualified in anything, he was once coincidently poised to relocate George II's dislocated thumb, an event that proved a perfect testimonial for the poison he claimed cured everything, including gout, scurvy and syphilis (three of the period's biggest afflictions). All it really did was make people sweat. James Morrison, soon after, amassed a fortune with his 'Vegetable Pills', the correct dose of which was 'as many pills as possible'. Unhappily they contained mostly purgatives and *The Lancet* medical journal published numerous reports of deaths, often due to excessive bowel movements. One London grocer swore to have taken 18,000 pills.

This was also the age of electricity. Galvani had sent it through frogs' legs, and thence electricity was seen as a life-giving force, a restorer of health. This, at least, was the belief of Franz Mesmer (1743–1815), who set up an elaborate Parisian establishment where patients sat holding hands around a wooden tub of liquid, iron filings and glass powder. Metal rods projected from the tub that healed ailing parts of the body. A glass harmonica played soothingly from behind astrologically patterned curtains, before Mesmer stepped out in a long purple robe and touched everyone with a white wand, a touch said to enhance the magnetic potency of the 'universal fluid'.

Those uncured by electricity could be assuaged by water, coming back in fashion as a means of becoming cured (though not as a means of becoming clean). In 1702 Queen Anne had visited Bath for treatment of gout, and spa towns soon sprouted everywhere, while coastal towns boasted the therapeutic properties of seawater (though peculiarly only seawater adjacent to the coastal town promoting it). An avid proponent was Dr Richard Russell (1687–1759), who in 1750 wrote *A Dissertation Concerning the Use of*

Sea-Water in Diseases of the Glands. In it he recommended seawater for almost any malady he cared to mention – and he was careful to mention many – and those affected were advised not just to immerse themselves in it but to drink it liberally. Seawater became so popular for everything from gout and jaundice to 'melancholy' and 'windiness' that, after Russell set up practice, his little coastal village saw influxes of people flocking to be relieved. One day that village would become Brighton. Tobias Smollett, novelist and doctor, took immersion overseas, to Nice, where he swam daily, something those in Nice contemplated curiously since the water had always been deemed too cold. But his subsequent writings did much to vitalize the future Riviera.

James Graham (1745–94), a self-proclaimed physician, 'specialized' in sexual dissatisfaction. His favoured devices were, rather alarmingly, water and electricity, thankfully not in quite sufficient proximity to make sexual dissatisfaction the least concern of his clients. Graham touted longevity and sexual rejuvenation for all who visited his Temple of Health off the Strand and partook in his milk or mud baths. Around about magnets and vibrating devices added uniquely to the experience, while music and perfume filled the air and ladies wandered about without clothes (including Amy Lyon, the future Lady Emma Hamilton, Nelson's mistress). Where bathing and nudity failed to cure ills or provide sexual agreeableness, Graham could offer, for £50 a night, his electrified 'Celestial Bed'.

Quacks were just as industrious in America. British medicines, including John Hooper's 'Female Pills' for 'young women afflicted with the irregularities' (one of the first patented medicines), were imported and popularized by newspapers (one reason quackery thrived). And apothecaries replenished old bottles with anything, no law demanding a drug be safe, far less effective.

Back in England, Graham's ideas became distinctly odder. His new therapy, 'earth-bathing', was unveiled in 1786, when Graham gave public exhibitions in which he lectured buried to his neck in earth. He began diverting his enthusiasm from eroticism to longevity. One of his lectures, *How to Live for Many Weeks or Months or Years Without Eating Anything Whatever*, proffered an impossible premise, followed unstoppably but received no less incredulously by his guarantee to audiences of healthy living to age 150.

▶ Hunter and surgery

The appeal of surgical anatomy, since Vesalius, at least on the deceased, never ceased. Dutch botanist Frederik Ruysch kept a large gallery of preserved body parts decorated with plants and coral. Peter the Great dissected his wife on her death, seemingly from curiosity. And in 1788 a Mrs Dodwell was acquitted of adultery when it emerged that Mr Edward Dodwell, an amateur anatomist, had a habit of dissecting cadavers in their bedroom.

Less dubiously, surgery in Edinburgh was highly regarded, and a great age of surgery was beginning. John Hunter (1728–93) set up his own anatomy school and surgical practice. In 1765 he bought a house near Earl's Court in London, with large grounds which housed a collection of animals (including zebra, Asiatic buffaloes, mountain goats and jackals). Here, on animals that died, he created his delicate dissections, with the finest of nerves displayed, astounding in precision.

Hunter was elected to the Royal Society in 1767, and considered the authority on venereal diseases, believing gonorrhoea and syphilis to be caused by a single pathogen. In an age when physicians often experimented on themselves, he inoculated himself with gonorrhoea with a needle unknowingly contaminated with syphilis. When reacting to both diseases, he claimed it proved his erroneous theory. Such was his reputation, the notion would not be disproved for half a century.

In 1768 Hunter was appointed surgeon to St George's Hospital, and in 1776 to King George III. In 1783 he moved to a large house in Leicester Square, with space to arrange his collection of 14,000 preparations of over 500 plant and animal species into a teaching museum. His was the first giraffe specimen ever to be seen in England, exciting the greatest interest. Also in 1783, in keeping with his apparent passion for knowledge of tall things, Hunter acquired the skeleton of a 7 ft 7 in (2 m 31 cm) Irishman named Charles Byrne, against Byrne's clear deathbed wishes to be buried at sea. Hunter bribed a member of the funeral party and filled the coffin with rocks, retrieving Byrne's body and subsequently publishing a description of his anatomy. Byrne's remains remain in the Hunterian Museum at the Royal College of Surgeons.

In 1786 Hunter was appointed deputy surgeon to the British Army, and in 1790 Surgeon General. He died in 1793 following an argument then a heart attack. That Hunter achieved wide respect is without doubt. That Hunter was often wrong is true. As well as his error with syphilis (possibly leading to his acquiring its cerebral complications), Hunter claimed that black Africans were white at birth, and that over time the sun turned skin black (he also claimed white blisters and burns on black skin evidence of white ancestry). That Hunter's ethics were dubious is debatable, but he was said to be kind to animals, self-sacrificing to patients and zealous in helping colleagues, and to the poor his services were rendered without remuneration. That Hunter was an eccentric appears incontestable. That Hunter was pivotal in promoting scientific enquiry is clear.

In the eighteenth century, drawing teeth, lancing boils and cutting syphilitic chancres were about the most enthralling things that could be done surgically (that patients could survive) although Claudius Aymand (1681–1740) is credited with the first successful appendectomy. Bloodletting, based on the notion that blood created disease, was still practised widely, as was cupping to suck blood and boils. But the surgeon's role was set to rise relentlessly. A superior method for removing bladder stones was performed by William Cheselden (1688–1752), who had already restored vision with cataract surgery. Cheselden operated with rapidity, a blessing. To make the transition to the modern era, surgery had yet to solve three critical problems: pain, infection and bleeding. Jean-Louis Petit (1674–1750), a French military surgeon, solved the latter with vascular tourniquets allowing thigh amputation. He also performed the first mastectomy. France would become a leading light in surgery.

With the rise in private anatomy schools and an academic basis developing, surgeons sought professional recognition, disuniting from barbers to form the Company of Surgeons in 1745. In 1800, granted Royal Charter, it became The Royal College of Surgeons. Its new building would house the Hunterian Collection.

Expanding surgical practice, with speed of the essence, and speed demanding anatomical familiarity, spawned a new problem: grave-robbing. Lack of refrigeration meant that corpses putrefied quickly, and with a constant need for fresh ones, graveyards were rich pastures for robbers to furrow. Many families held on to the bodies of departed loved ones until they rotted and lost their value, while graveyards employed armed watchmen. All of which made some robbers switch to the safer method of murder. William Burke and William Hare began their routine of getting wastrels drunk and suffocating them in November 1827; they took bodies repeatedly to Professor Robert

Knox in Edinburgh, who paid between £7 and £14 a corpse. Surely suspicious, he elected to say nothing, although his career was ruined once the scandal emerged. Hare escaped hanging by agreeing to testify against Burke, but Burke made a full confession and was swiftly hanged. His body was made available to Alexander Monro, grandson of the medical school's founder, and bits were made into keepsakes (including a purse) still in museums today. Charles Darwin (1809–82) had been Monro's student just two years earlier, but finding lectures dull and surgery distressing, pursued a different course.

▶ Lind's medical research and Jenner's vaccination

In 1747, off the Bay of Biscay, James Lind (1716–94), a Royal Navy doctor of less incurious disposition than many peers investigated, among many things, the advantages of clean quarters. His inquisitive mind also led him to discover that eating fruit treated and prevented scurvy. Most notable about Lind's investigation was not that he discovered scurvy's cause, but that he divided 12 scurvy sufferers into six groups and exposed different groups to different interventions, a landmark method that would one day lead to the most robust means of studying treatment-effect in modern medicine, the randomized controlled trial. Those given two oranges and a lemon each day recovered most – if you'll forgive the choice of word – fruitfully.

A little later, in sleepy villages in England, milkmaids were going about their business. Edward Jenner (1749–1823), no less enquiring than Lind, and friend of John Hunter, was contemplating something else. Jenner was a vicar's son in the Gloucestershire village of Berkeley, a nature-lover writing such verses as *Address to a Robin*. He practised medicine in his birthplace, for city life never appealed, nor fortune. The idea of vaccination was conveyed to him by a dairymaid's remark, 'I can't take smallpox, for I have already had cowpox'. Cowpox was a relatively mild disease, with blisters transmitted from the udder of the cow to the hands of the milker, and it was generally known in Gloucestershire that the milkmaid's statement was true. Smallpox was an indiscriminately deadly and disfiguring disease. Elizabeth I was nearly killed by it, but recovered completely. Her friend Lady Mary Sidney became, wrote her husband, 'as foul a lady as the smallpox could make her'. A century later Frances Stuart, Duchess of Richmond, who modelled as Britannia for the English penny and was said to be unfailingly beautiful, was profoundly disfigured (though to the unwavering affections of Charles II).

On 14 May 1796 Jenner 'vaccinated' eight-year-old James Phipps with pus from the hand of a milkmaid, Sarah Nelmes, who was infected with cowpox. Eight weeks later Jenner inoculated the boy with smallpox. No disease appeared. The rest, as they say, is history, and Jenner, immune himself to the illuminations of fame, remained a

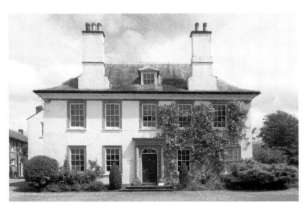

▲ Figure 8.1 Edward Jenner's home.

village doctor, fossil collector and fruit-grower, and, amid his cuckoos and hedgehogs, vaccinated the poor in an arbour of his garden.

Smallpox emerged in the Middle East perhaps 6,000–10,000 years ago, provoking fear, scientific interest and malign intention throughout history. Smallpox was first used as a biological weapon by the British in the French and Indian wars of 1754–67, blankets from infected patients being distributed to American Indians whose population was halved. In the American War of Independence (1775–83) the British tried the ploy again, this time with blankets containing scabs and skin-flakes from disease victims wafted via riders on horseback through enemy camps at night. The ploy was (in part) foiled by the foresight of George Washington who had ordered 'vaccination' of his armies. While vaccination methods were amateur (troops were encouraged to wander close to victims and even lie down in their bedding) the strategy seems to have been effective. Many of Washington's men died of smallpox, but enough survived to assure victory and the founding of a nation.

Jenner's preventive medicine, and Lind's method of determining best treatment, would help push medicine towards an altogether new era.

The Ages Between 'Early Modern' and Modern Medicine: Nineteenth-Century Medicine

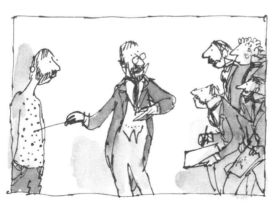

9

The Age of Hospitals and Physicians

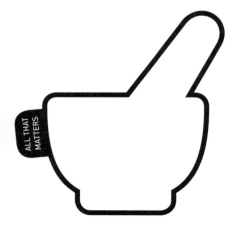

▶ The rise of hospitals, clinical medicine and bedside teaching

Hospitals had proliferated in the 1700s, largely charitable, run by religious orders. The first in London were the Westminster (1720), Guy's (1724), St George's (1733), the London (1740) and the Middlesex (1745). Edinburgh Royal Infirmary opened in 1729, followed by hospitals in Winchester and Bristol (1737), York (1740), Exeter (1741), Bath (1742) and other provincial cities such that by 1800 every sizeable town had one and 20,000 patients went through their doors annually. Britain was behind the rest of Europe, already building bigger hospitals – such as Vienna's 2,000-bed Allgemeines Krankenhaus (1784), Berlin's Charité (1768) and St Petersburg's Obukhov Hospital – but ahead of North America where the first was in Philadelphia (1751), followed 20 years later by the New York Hospital and the Massachusetts General in 1811. A hundred years later America would have over 4,000. Early 'lying-in' or maternity hospitals took root, although it was undoubtedly safer to undergo labour at home. Before 1800 hospitals offered mostly food, shelter and rest. They were crowded, and infections thrived there.

Transforming hospitals into anything resembling today's institutions would be slow, but a number of things came together in the nineteenth century. Medical science advanced. Teaching became aligned to hospitals, where professors with clinical beds instructed on cases. And physicians viewed hospitals no longer as places of convalescence but as places of real medical business, where patients were treated and students taught. Paris led the way in this 'clinical' medicine, pioneered by René Théophile Hyacinthe Laënnec (1781–1826), inventor of the stethoscope and physician at the Necker and the Pitié-Salpêtrière hospitals, and Pierre-Charles-Alexandre Louis (1787–72) at the Hôtel-Dieu. The 'clinic', as hospital medicine came to be called, was the setting for hands-on examination of patients, observation by students on ward rounds and the correlation of the outward manifestations of disease with the inner pathology. Post-mortem examinations shifted to hospitals, the wards and morgue ideal for students to flit between.

The nineteenth century also brought the first specialist hospitals that offered more good than harm: the Royal Hospital for Diseases of the Chest (1814); the Brompton Hospital for tuberculosis (1841); the Royal Marsden Hospital for cancer (1851); the Hospital for Sick Children, Great Ormond Street (1852); and the National Hospital, Queen Square, for nervous diseases (1860). Children's hospitals emerged in Paris (Hôpital des Enfants-Malades, 1802, on the site of an orphanage), Berlin, Vienna and St Petersburg. North America sprouted the Massachusetts Eye and Ear Infirmary, the Boston Lying-In Hospital and the New York Hospital for Diseases of the Skin. Expansion and diversification of hospitals would now be unstoppable.

▶ Cholera and public health

On 3 September 1878, the pleasure boat *Princess Alice*, overflowing with day-trippers after a day at the seaside, was returning to London up the River Thames. She collided with an 890-ton collier and sank in four minutes, with many trapped inside. The twice-daily release of 75 million imperial gallons (340 million litres) of raw sewage from outfalls at Barking and Crossness had occurred an hour before; the heavily polluted water claimed the lives of many escaping the boat. Over 650 drowned in sludge, and corpses bobbed to the surface for days, many so bloated from bacterial gases they could not fit into coffins. The new sewage outfalls contributed to the greatest tragedy on the

Thames, but the outfalls were the result of a nineteenth-century scourge new to Britain.

Cholera, its name derived from its relentless watery stools, would rage in three pandemics during the nineteenth century. The first, beginning in 1812, was largely confined to Asia. The second began in 1829 and just reached Europe, introducing a disease whose dehydration with 'blue lips' and 'shrivelled hollow face' could kill in less than a day. The third came in the middle of the century. The year 1854 proved a devastating one.

In the mid-1800s, people obtained water from communal wells and pumps. And in London, water from the Thames was ferried to breweries and businesses. Meanwhile, most sewage was dumped directly into open 'cesspits' or, more commonly, the Thames (which also received offal, dead animals, industrial waste and anything else unwanted). Toilets were still in their infancy, and cellars of houses were often filled with human waste many feet deep; outside brick stepping-stones were often assembled across feculent yards.

John Harrington is credited with the first flush toilet, installing one for his godmother Queen Elizabeth I. By all accounts she loved it, though by most accounts it wasn't very good. Joseph Bramah had patented the modern flush toilet in 1778, but these – for those who could afford one – often unsavourily backfired from cesspits and sewers. The dilemma would be dissipated by the deliberations of Thomas Crapper, devising a U-bend with water trap and elevated cistern, the pull of a chain activating a rush of swirling and altogether more savoury water taking things away for good. So far, so good. Except that in 1854 Crapper was but 18 years old, yet to invent his aforementioned toilet (and yet to be erroneously associated with the word 'crap', a word with far more distant origins). But even had Crapper's toilets been around in 1854, most sewers were designed for rainwater, not anything solid.

All of which set the stage comfortably for cholera when it arrived in Britain.

Cholera evoked little fear at first, not because it wasn't rampant but because it ravaged the poor. As the state medical commission in New York declared when it first struck that city, it 'arises entirely from their habits of life'. Only when cholera struck well-to-do neighbourhoods did it become a national obsession. Between 1845 and 1856, over 700 works on cholera were published in London, none answering the most pressing question of all: What was it? 'What is cholera?' *The Lancet* asked in 1853. 'Is it a fungus, an insect, a miasma, an electrical disturbance, a deficiency of ozone, a morbid off-scouring of the intestinal canal? We know nothing.' The most prevalent thought was that cholera mysteriously and invisibly lingered in impure air. Anything foul – sewage, offal, a corpse – was felt to add to the 'impure air' in which cholera thrived, and the more air smelt, the more deadly it was felt to be.

There was one serious disbeliever in this 'miasma' theory: John Snow (1813–58). Snow studied medicine in Newcastle before becoming an anaesthetist in London. Anaesthesia was still in its infancy with only chloroform available, a decidedly dangerous chemical if the person administering it decided on the wrong dose and as there was no known right dose, administering the wrong dose was all too frequent. And so when in 1853 Snow administered chloroform to Queen Victoria in labour in her eighth pregnancy, with Leopold, he was considered at best incautious (though Snow would go on to attend her ninth labour, with Beatrice, just a week after experimenting with other anaesthetic agents with fatal consequence). But Snow was the first to apply dose calculation in anaesthesia, and so led to its greater safety.

But it was not Snow's anaesthetic sojourns that would provide his enduring legacy. It was what he did in 1854.

Snow was an unusual doctor. He considered that poverty created the conditions for disease rather than that disease originated in poor people. He saw a serious flaw in the miasma theory, too: Cholera devastated parts of London while sparing others: in Southwark, death rates were six times greater than neighbouring Lambeth, and if cholera was caused by bad air, then why would people breathing the same air display such discordant infection rates? Snow believed that there was a link between cholera and water contaminated with sewage, a belief heightened in August 1854 when Soho was affected with unprecedented fury. 'Within 250 yards of the spot where Cambridge Street joins Broad Street there were upwards of 500 fatal attacks of cholera in 10 days,' Snow wrote. 'I suspected some contamination of the water of the much-frequented street-pump in Broad Street.' Besides those living near the pump, he tracked hundreds of cholera cases to nearby schools and businesses. One café-owner serving water from the Broad Street pump declared that nine customers had cholera. Snow also investigated groups spared from cholera. A workhouse prison near Soho had virtually no cases. Snow discovered it had its own well. A brewery on Broad Street escaped. It, too, had its own well. One victim died in Hampstead and another in Islington – miles away from Broad Street. Snow discovered that the Hampstead victim enjoyed the Broad Street water so much she had it delivered to her home, while the Islington victim, her niece, had visited for tea.

On 7 September 1854, Snow persuaded the parish council to remove the handle from the Broad Street pump. But he met strong resistance when he appeared before a parliamentary select committee, the chairman asking, 'Are the Committee to understand ... that no matter how offensive to the sense of smell the effluvia ... you consider that it is not prejudicial in any way to the health of the inhabitants of the district?'

Snow was often at best disliked. Edwin Chadwick, Poor Law reformer and author of *A Report on the Sanitary Condition of the Labouring Population*, believed heartedly that getting rid of smells got rid of disease. 'All smell is disease', he explained to a parliamentary inquiry. *The Lancet* concluded that Snow was vested by businesses wishing to fill the air with 'pestilent vapours, miasms and loathsome abominations of every kind', and the parliamentary committee told Snow, 'we see no reason to adopt this belief'.

Undeterred, Snow continued tracing almost all cases of cholera to the Broad Street pump, including children using it en route to school. What Snow couldn't prove was the outbreak's source. This information would come from an unlikely aid, the Reverend Henry Whitehead, a local curate who had contended cholera came from God's divine intervention. But Whitehead must have been sufficiently open-minded and magnanimous to agree 'slowly, and I may add reluctantly, that the use of water was connected with the continuation of the outburst'. Whitehead then interviewed a woman living in Broad Street whose baby had contracted cholera elsewhere, and who dumped her baby's nappy water into a leaky cesspool three feet from the Broad Street pump.

John Snow died quietly from a stroke in June 1858. Today, he is considered the pioneer of public health. His epidemiological maps showing the exact distributions of cholera victims are among the most important documents in the history of public health. Edwin Chadwick died in 1890, 14 years after a microbial cause of cholera was identified. He never stopped believing that smells caused disease, continuing until his death to propose ways of dissipating smells to make disease disappear. One was to erect a series of towers (modelled on Paris's new Eiffel Tower) that would act as mighty ventilators, pulling in healthy air from the heights and pumping it out at the ground.

Summer 1858 found London in a heatwave. 'The Great Stink', as *The Times* dubbed it, made it apparent that London needed new sewers, a formidable task that fell to Joseph Bazalgette (1819–91). His excavations would redistribute 3.5 million cubic yards of earth, creating 1,200 miles of tunnels from 318 million bricks, and the three three-and-a-half miles of Chelsea, Albert and Victoria riverfront embankments narrowing the river. Bazalgette's system still drains London today. With limited budget, he could take sewage only as far as the eastern edge of the city, to Barking. There, mighty outfalls discharged 150 million gallons of sewage into the Thames each day. Something of great solace to the people of London.

Something of great sorrow to all aboard *Princess Alice* on her fateful day in 1878.

▶ Osler, expanding clinical methods and teaching

In 1831 Featherstone Osler, born in Falmouth, Cornwall, grandson of a pirate, was invited to serve as science officer on *HMS Beagle*. A former Royal Navy Lieutenant serving on *HMS Victory*, he declined Darwin's voyage as his father was dying, and pursued a sedentary life. He fathered William Osler in Canada in 1849.

William Osler (1849–1919) would become the first Physician-in-Chief at Johns Hopkins Hospital in Baltimore in 1889. He was one of Johns Hopkins's 'big four' founding professors: Osler, Professor of Medicine; William Halsted, Professor of Surgery; Howard Kelly, Professor of

Gynaecology; and William Welch, Professor of Pathology. Osler promoted medicine as an eloquent science, drawing on all knowledge of diagnostics and therapeutics to date, and urged students to the bedside. 'He who studies medicine without books sails an uncharted sea, but he who studies medicine without patients does not go to sea at all' was one of his best known sayings, but perhaps more important was his ethos of the patient being central in the practice of medicine. 'Listen to your patient, he is telling you the diagnosis', he would say, emphasizing the importance of taking a good history and respect for the patient. Humanity he had in abundance. Once handing a beggar his overcoat, he added, 'You may drink yourself to death, but I cannot allow you to freeze to death'.

Osler's approach encapsulated an important transformation in the medical profession during the nineteenth century. Traditionally, physicians, unlike surgeons, were largely 'hands off': what mattered were scholarly judgement and bedside manner. Upon diagnosis they formulated a regimen, often herbal, prepared by an apothecary. Physicians were considered learned and upstanding, and better with age. Through the nineteenth century, physicians became more 'hands on' and clinical signs became valued information. Eponymous signs and diseases still abound in medicine, and many names came from this era: Richard Bright, Thomas Addison, Robert Graves, William Stokes, Dominic Corrigan, Armand Trousseau and Adolph Kussmaul, to name but a few. The stethoscope (for auscultation, listening to internal sounds) had been introduced in 1816. The ophthalmoscope (for eye examination) and laryngoscope (for throat examination) now appeared, as did compact thermometers and sphygmomanometers (for measuring blood pressure). Paris, Edinburgh, London, Dublin, Vienna and Strasbourg were among famous centres of medicine.

A revolution in medical education was inextricably linked to physicians. New medical schools arose, older ones were transformed and intakes grew. By the mid-1800s education was not solely about morals and values. Students everywhere – North America included – returned from France equipped with knowledge of pathology, physiology, chemistry and cells – and carried a stethoscope to prove their worth. From the 1830s, London had a medical university with two colleges, University and King's, with purpose-built hospitals. By 1840 St Bartholomew's had 300 students. Vienna's clinical medicine, particularly, illuminated the era. A typical curriculum of the 1880s included zoology, mineralogy, botany, chemistry, physiology, anatomy, pathology, pharmacology, therapy, bandages and instruments, forensic medicine, vaccination, toxicology, formulary and veterinary medicine. Medical journals like *The New England Journal of Medicine* (est. 1812) and *The Lancet* (est. 1823) helped disperse knowledge.

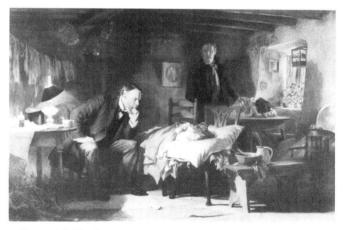

▲ Figure 9.1 The Doctor. Luke Fildes, 1891.

Quacks thrived in the eighteenth century, while the nineteenth brought anti-orthodox ideas to counter physicians in the forms of homeopathy, hydrotherapy, osteopathy and chiropractice (the latter's founder Daniel Palmer claimed to have restored a man's hearing by spinal manipulation).

In the meantime, articles penned by Dr Egerton Yorrick Davis, a retired US Army surgeon living in Quebec, seemed authoritative. In an 1884 issue of *Philadelphia Medical News*, Yorrick Davis described 'an uncommon form of vaginismus'. A maid engaged in sexual intercourse had experienced severe vaginal spasm, her coachman lover unable to 'remove himself'. Yorrick Davis reported having relaxed and separated the couple with chloroform, naming the condition 'penis captivus'. Yorrick Davis was also an avid attendee of events and conferences, sometimes signing in with William Osler's wife. It would soon become clear that Yorrick Davis and William Osler were one, that the army surgeon's articles were factitious, as indeed was he.

Soon afterwards, Osler would be Regius Professor of Medicine at Oxford.

Make of that what you will.

10

The Age of
Antiseptics and
Anaesthetics

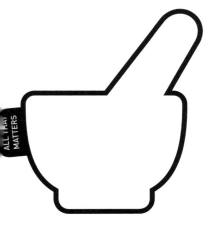

ALL THAT
MATTERS

▶ The laboratory comes of age

The 'school' of nineteenth-century Parisian physicians, nucleated in hospitals, would spark something extraordinary: a sort of allied but rival institution, the laboratory.

Bichat's legacy found support in François-Joseph-Victor Broussais (1772–1838), who argued that his contemporaries lingered much on pathological anatomy, but should dwell more on disease processes.

Laboratories were not new. Hooke and Boyle had pioneered an experimentation age, but nineteenth-century physiologists, chemists and microscopists felt that, while hospitals were for healing, the laboratory would be where things could be rigorously tested under controlled conditions.

Justus von Liebig (1803–73) developed an Institute of Chemistry at the University of Giessen in Germany with unparalleled devotion to his subject. Liebig invented a silvering process to make mirrors. He discovered he could concentrate yeast, making Marmite's precursor. And he was first to subject living organisms to strict experimentation, measuring what went in (food, water, oxygen) and what came out (urea, salts and acids, carbon dioxide) and developing a notion of metabolic processes driving life. He inaugurated biochemistry.

Germany would dominate physiology, too. Johannes Müller's *Handbook of Physiology* (in two vast volumes, something peculiar about handbooks) would serve generations. In later life Müller became ever-intrigued by fish and marine life, authored a comprehensive work on the anatomy of amphibians and described several new species of snake. But notwithstanding Müller's deviation from physiology, he had encouraged many physiologist protégés: Hermann von Helmholtz, Emil du Bois-Reymond, Carl Ludwig, Ernst Wilhelm von Brücke, Theodor Schwann and Friedrich Gustav Jakob Henle to name but a few. Helmholtz, Bois-Reymond, Ludwig and Brücke committed to explaining life in physico-chemical ways through experimental physiology. Helmholtz elevated nerve conduction's understanding to new heights, invented the ophthalmoscope (1850) and was curious about the brain's response to aesthetics, the visual world and music. Bois-Reymond spent much of his life examining nerve and muscle electrophysiology, and in 1880 spoke to the Berlin Academy of Sciences outlining seven 'world riddles', some of which neither science nor philosophy would ever explain, including the origins of life, sensation and thought. Ludwig is best remembered for deducing how urine is made, but should perhaps be known for his insistence that animal experiments be undertaken with utmost care to avoid inflicting pain (through anaesthetic) and that deductions had full scientific value. Brücke is best remembered for leaving for Vienna and as Freud's role model.

From 1830 the microscope became a more advanced instrument. In 1838 Schwann extended cell theory, restricted largely to plants since Hooke, to animals. Then cell theory was elaborated into a theory of disease by German pathologist Rudolf Virchow (1821–1902), professor of anatomy at Berlin who did for the cell what Bichat had done for tissues; in *Die Cellularpathologie* (1858) he asserted that all cells originated from cells, and that all disease was a disease of cells.

France had created a new era of hospitals, but by the mid-1800s Germany dominated laboratory science. But one Frenchman, a failed dramatist, made his mark. Claude Bernard (1813–78) sought 'to establish the use of the scientific method in medicine'. He is most associated with the concept of 'milieu intérieur' or homeostasis (the internal environment's constancy), though he studied poisons with passion, devoted particularly to curare and carbon monoxide. Bernard was the primary proponent of vivisection of his time, with the rational: 'the physiologist is no ordinary man. He is a learned man, a man possessed and absorbed by a scientific idea. He does not hear the animals' cries of pain. He is blind to the blood that flows.' It was all too much for his wife and daughter, unconvinced the advancement of medicine justified such suffering of animals, and his wife left him in 1869 to campaign against it. Physician George Hoggan, after spending time in Bernard's laboratory, had similar misgivings, and became 'prepared to see not only science, but even mankind, perish rather than have recourse to such means of saving it'.

Scientific medicine arose more slowly in North America, but Johns Hopkins, its major medical institution (and the only school to admit women) prized teaching and research and its illuminaries inaugurated the Rockefeller Institute for Medical Research in New York in 1901.

Britain lagged behind yet further scientifically, winning its place ultimately in physiology in Edinburgh and Cambridge. But Britain's 1876 Cruelty to Animals Act, stipulating how animals should be treated, would be matched by no nation until well into the twentieth century.

▶ Germs

Louis Pasteur (1822–95) was a Parisian chemist. An outstanding microscopist, he observed that maggots arose from insect-laid eggs, and that many organisms are invisible to the naked eye (so much so that he developed a habit of taking a microscope to meals). His interest in micro-organisms was fermented, so to speak, by fermenting wine and beer.

The cause – aetiology – of infectious diseases until now had been controversial. The two main theories were miasma (effluvia and other emanations from earth and atmosphere) and contagion (spread from person to person, though nobody knew how).

Germ theory would take the world by storm, Pasteur at its epicentre, although the idea wasn't new, and the microscope had long revealed the pervasive presence of a miniature world all around us. Pasteur, however, was first to show that microbes could cause disease, in cows, pigs and poultry, and then in humans.

Pasteur was interested in practicality, in the therapeutic potentials of science, surprisingly lacking so far in a world devoted to science for at least two centuries. His research on chicken cholera, anthrax and erysipelas would lead to 'vaccines', a term derived from Jenner's cowpox inoculation against smallpox (*vacca* Latin for cow), using the principle of priming the body's defences with exposure to attenuated or lesser forms of the disease.

In spectacular experiments, Pasteur had no equal. In April 1881 he injected 24 sheep with his anthrax vaccine, repeating it three weeks later. A fortnight later he injected the 24 animals, and a further control group not primed with vaccine, with live anthrax. By June, all vaccinated sheep were healthy, all unvaccinated sheep dead. He developed other vaccines, and his method of eliminating harmful micro-organisms from milk, pasteurization, would eliminate milk as a source of tuberculosis and other disease.

Robert Koch (1843–1910), a German contemporary of Pasteur, later professor of public health in Berlin, postulated the conditions necessary to prove a particular microbe caused a particular disease, and famously discovered *Bacillus anthracis* (1876), *Mycobacterium tuberculosis* (1882) and *Vibrio cholerae* (1883).

Fatal epidemics were commonplace in the pre-antibiotic world. Tick-borne typhus replaced syphilis as the scourge of ill-kempt soldiers, and thwarted Napoleon's invasion of Russia. Typhoid ('like typhus' because it produced a similar lethargy, although an altogether different disease) would kill more soldiers in the Boer War battles than combat. Prince Albert would die of it. Mary Mallon ('Typhoid Mary') was the first person identified as an asymptomatic carrier of it, infecting and unknowingly killing countless in her career as a cook. Bursts of measles, diphtheria, influenza, rheumatic fever, scarlet fever and smallpox, among other infectious diseases, killed many more.

Knowing the enemy would be half the battle, and Pasteur and Koch opened the gates to identifying causal microbes for typhoid, diphtheria, streptococcal pneumonia, meningococcal meningitis, brucellosis (undulant fever), gonorrhoea, syphilis, tetanus, leprosy, plague and many, many more.

The other half of the battle would be treating them.

▶ Painless, clean surgery

One of the easiest ways to die, still, was to undergo surgery. And those who didn't die sometimes wished they had.

In 1806 English novelist Fanny Burney, living in Paris, suffered pain in her right breast. The problem was diagnosed as breast cancer and a mastectomy was ordered, a job for Napoleon's surgeon-in-chief, Baron Dominique-Jean Larrey (1766–1842), famed for low mortality rates and high speed (after the Battle of Borodino he managed 200 amputations in 24 hours), something of the essence since anaesthesia was still some years off. Burney's apprehension was furious, heightened by her surgeon's delay. As the clock struck three, seven grave men in black entered the room. A bed was

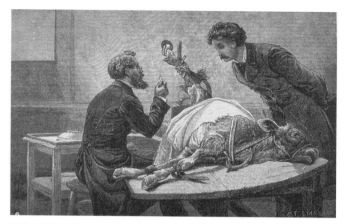

▲ Figure 10.1 Vaccination from the Calf. Charles Joseph Staniland, 1883. National Library of Medicine.

moved to the middle, but 'nothing clean so as not to spoil good linen'. A handkerchief was placed over her face.

In her diary, she later wrote: 'When the dreadful steel was plunged into the breast – cutting through veins – arteries – flesh – nerves – I needed no injunctions not to restrain my cries. I began a scream ... I almost marvel that it rings not in my ears still, so excruciating was the agony. When the wound was made, and the instrument was withdrawn, the pain seemed undiminished, for the air that suddenly rushed into those delicate parts felt like a mass of minute but sharp and forked poniards, that were tearing the edges of the wound ... when again I felt the instrument ... cutting against the grain ... while the flesh resisted in a manner so forcible as to oppose and tire the hand of the operator ...presently the terrible cutting was renewed – and worse than ever, to separate the bottom, the foundation of this dreadful gland from the parts to which it adhered ... I then felt the knife tackling against the breast bone – scraping it!'

The procedure lasted seventeen-and-a-half minutes. It took Burney months to recover. But she lived another 29 years, suggesting that the lump may have been benign.

Surgery was daring, often deadly, and dreadful for those subjected to it. Amputations were normally performed in less than a minute, but vessels still had to be tied off and wounds sutured. Unsurprisingly, people were often driven to attempt home remedies. Gouverneur Morris, one of the signatories of the Declaration of Independence, killed himself by forcing whalebone into his penis trying to clear a blockage.

Before anaesthesia, ways to lessen pain included bleeding patients to the point of faintness (often causing death), alcohol, opium, hashish and, not infrequently, albeit always ineffectually, infusing tobacco into the rectum. Thus when William Clarke (1819–98) in Rochester assisted a tooth extraction with ether in January 1842, Crawford Long (1815–78) removed a neck tumour with it in the same year, and five years later London surgeon Robert Liston (1794–1847) used it to amputate a limb, it marked the beginning of operations that could venture where they never had before, and would revolutionize surgical practice.

In 1772 Joseph Priestley (1733–1804) discovered nitrous oxide. Soon afterwards Humphry Davy (1778–1829) from Penzance coined it 'laughing gas', discovering its anaesthetic properties with Bristol physician Thomas Beddoes (1760–1808). Chemistry was becoming decidedly practical. Ether would later prove more effective, and then chloroform, judged to be safer.

Post-operative death rates remained shockingly high, however, from septicaemia (blood poisoning from infection). Joseph Lister (1827–1912) would eventually respond to this call, but Ignaz Semmelweis (1818–65), an often forgotten Hungarian physician working in the Vienna Allgemeines Krankenhaus maternity wards, should be remembered for his observation that death rates in mothers (from puerperal fever) were staggeringly higher in births conducted by 'medical men' than by midwives. He theorized that medical staff and students, who went straight from the mortuary to the delivery suite without washing their hands, were vectors of disease. In 1847 he urged hand and instrument washing with chlorinated lime solution and demonstrated that mortality rates dropped to levels seen in midwives' clinics. Unhappily, Semmelweis's contemporaries were unconvinced by his results (germ theory not yet being established). Semmelweis could not explain his findings scientifically and died, in a lunatic asylum, ironically from septicaemia through a finger-cut.

As late as 1861 Dr Harriet Austin would write a book called *Baths and How to Take Them*. But views on personal sanitation were, thankfully, changing. Oddly, as Victorians switched from scepticism about washing to comfort in the notion, and theories about personal hygiene were reversed (dirty people – Thackeray's great unwashed – were so often sick) it took time for surgeons to accept the idea.

Antiseptics were not unknown (wine, vinegar and iodine were known to counter putrefaction), but it was Lister who put antiseptic techniques into surgery. Lister was professor of surgery at Glasgow Royal Infirmary in 1861 when he believed carbolic acid might be effective antisepsis, trialling it on 11-year-old James Greenlees whose leg had been run over by a cart resulting in an open tibial fracture. The wound healed perfectly, convincing Lister to develop antiseptic practice and publish his conclusion in *The Lancet* in 1867 that germs caused disease and pus was bad, expanded in his *Antiseptic Principle of the Practice of Surgery*. Koch would soon urge heat sterilization of instruments, while Johns Hopkins surgeons started wearing rubber gloves. Lister, who sported long side-whiskers and was a friend of Pasteur, became surgical professor in Edinburgh. Despite his wife Lady Lister's death in 1893, he was thence persuaded to London, where antisepsis had made little headway. In 1895 he became President of the Royal Society.

Now surgeons could operate without restriction. Names like Theodore Billroth, Friedrich Trendelenburg and Theodore Kocher led the way in this new dawn, largely in abdominal surgery. Brothers William and Charles Mayo did the same in America. And Sir Rickman Godlee, Lister's nephew, was first to remove a brain tumour. By 1900 surgeons and operating theatres were respectively gowned and gleaming. By 1902 Edward VII's appendectomy (by Sir Frederick Treves) just before his coronation would go uneventfully.

Anaesthesia was well established. Antisepsis had come of age. And antibiotics were just around the corner.

11

The Age of 'Madness', Military Morbidity and Macabre Mortality

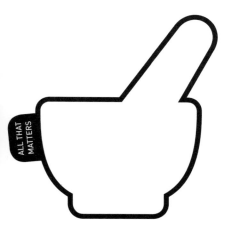

ALL THAT MATTERS

▶ 'Madness'

Psychiatry has distant origins. Bethlem Royal Hospital (Bedlam) in London dates from the thirteenth century. In 1758 William Battie's *Treatise on Madness* urged treatment in asylums and 30 years later, following King George III's remission from his then unknown condition porphyria, mental illness flickered in people's minds as something which might not be a life sentence. But in the 1700s members of the public could visit Bedlam, and for a penny peer into cells, view the 'freaks of the show' and laugh at them. Entry was free on the first Tuesday of the month. Nothing was known about mental illness, and through the 1800s hopeless cases were amassed into ever larger asylums.

Jewish-Austrian neurologist Sigmund Freud (1856–1939), inspired by physiology, took a different stance: a scientific one. Freud's psychoanalysis is now demoted as pseudoscience, and his prevailing view that just about every ill had a sexual element left many of his patients without cure. But he did help some by pointing out the obvious: 'Sometimes a cigar is just a cigar,' he once said. And one thing seems clear: Freud was one of the first to think mental illness curable.

▶ Military morbidity

Surgery was frequently advanced by battle. Baron Larry could amputate an unsalvageable leg (by the 'circular' method) in 13 seconds. But before anaesthetics, military medicine could but grumble along, and reconstructive surgery was incontemplatable.

In 1803 British military surgery became a special subject, directed by John Thomson (1765–1846). Yet in the Crimean War, 50 years later, there was still no sign of improved living conditions for soldiers, still plagued by infections,

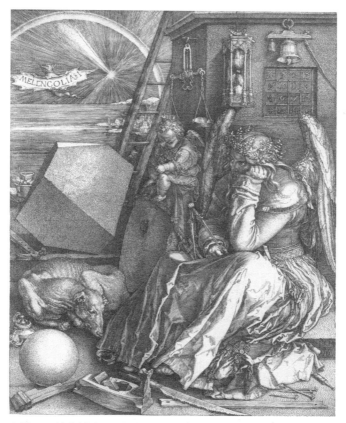

▲ Figure 11.1 Melencolia, Albrecht Dürer, 1514.

or of improved outcomes following injury. But in 1857, just after the Crimean War, and just before the Red Cross was established, an 'Army Hospital Corps' of specially trained men was formed to aid soldiers on and off the battlefield. In 1898 it received Queen Victoria's royal warrant, inaugurating the Royal Army Medical Corps.

By World War I, antisepsis and anaesthesia, and earlier treatment afforded by field hospitals and casualty clearing stations, considerably altered how the wounded suffered. Wholesale amputation was no longer needed. Typhoid vaccination almost eradicated this great infectious killer of the recent Boer War. But the Army Medical Department was faced with new problems, just as grave, occasioned by new weapons and new methods of warfare. Deaths from wound trauma now exceeded those from sepsis, injuries from shellfire providing new horrors and setting new challenges. Trench foot caused by prolonged exposure to wet, muddy terrain and trench fever, transmitted by body lice, were rife.

New wars, it seemed, merely brought new modes of death and disease.

▶ Macabre mortality

In the 1800s people had peculiar habits when it came to death. For one thing, they didn't always dispose of bodies, or body parts, and not for any scientific motive. In 1825 Artist William Brockedon visited a hospice on the Great St Bernard Pass in the Alps where a monk kept corpses in 'the postures in which they had perished'. In 1827 a book was bound with human skin. Then in 1839 the remains of thousands of bodies were found in a vault beneath Enon Chapel off London's Strand, the collection of its minister who promised that, for the bargain fee of 15 shillings, he could provide burials. To do this he crammed 12,000 bodies into a 12 ft × 59 ft (3.7 m × 18 m) pit over a period of 17 years. The 1852 Burial Act would outlaw such mischief.

But fear of being buried alive was rife among Victorians. Catalepsy, a condition of paralysis in which victims appeared dead, filled newspapers with terrifying tales. Eleanor Markham of upstate New York was being buried in July 1894 when anxious noises came from her coffin: 'I was conscious all the time you were making preparations to bury me,' she said on her extrication. 'The horror of my situation is altogether beyond description. I could hear everything that was going on.' Similar stories emerged everywhere; what seemed to evade everyone's consideration was that in all cases the paralysed, mute victim oddly regained movement and voice just when it mattered. Yet so many people were so obsessed with the fear of premature internment that arrangements were often made pre-empting it. In 1868 Hannah Beswick was finally buried, having paid Charles White, her physician, to examine her regularly after death for signs of life. White kept her embalmed body inside his grandfather clock, duly examining her annually until his death, when Beswick's body went into Manchester's Natural History Museum and thence the city's cemetery. In the same year Franz Vester in America devised a coffin with an escape hatch and ladder 'should a person be interred ere life is extinct'. Many directed that their heads be cut off before burial, to put things 'comfortably' to rest. Special mortuaries in Germany held corpses while they decomposed to a point they could be safely buried. Bodies were wired to bells designed to ring at the slightest movement, summoning porters to their aid. Usually the bell rang because of the gaseous bloating of decomposition.

Cremation, an alternative to burial that would solve the problem of populous bodies (and assuage the fears of those who might still be alive) was a long time coming, at least in Britain. William Price, Welsh doctor and fierce proponent, did little to advance it. A druid, he fathered a child in his eighties by his housekeeper and named it Jesus Christ. Believing burial damaging to the environment, when the baby died in 1883 he cremated it on a pyre on his land, where gathering villagers found him dancing in one of his costumes (he favoured a fox-head). Sir Henry Thompson, Queen Victoria's surgeon and founder of the Cremation Society of England, made a more persuasive case for cremation: 'it was becoming a necessary sanitary precaution', he said, having already demonstrated its efficacy by cremating a horse in his Woking ovens in 1879. In 1882 the family of Captain Thomas Hanham was cremated. The Home Secretary had refused the Cremation Society authority to dispose of Hanham's wife and mother, deceased respectively in 1876 and 1877, and Hanham eventually built his own crematorium in Dorset to do so. The verdict in Price's subsequent trial was that cremation was legal 'providing no nuisance is caused', leading to the first unhindered cremation at Woking, of Jeanette Pickersgill, on 26 March 1885. And Price, upon death, had his wishes granted, burning atop two tons of coal.

12

The Age of
Medical Women

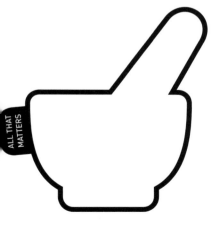

ALL THAT MATTERS

▶ The struggle for women

Until this point in history women had been misunderstood, marginalized and woefully maligned. The list of mistreatments is endlessly exhaustive. Rome's Vestal virgins were buried alive if they lost their virginity, while St Agatha of Sicily (patron saint of breast cancer) was placed in a brothel for 'retaining her virtue', with her breasts cut off. A Bill from the British Parliament in 1690 made it possible for a man to divorce a woman (and have her killed) on almost any grounds he saw fit, including her use of **'scents, paints, cosmetics, washes, artificial teeth, false hair, Spanish wool, iron stays, hoops, high-heeled shoes, or bolstered hips', incurring the penalty of 'laws now in force against witchcraft, sorcery, and such like misdemeanours'.** In 1832 Carlisle farmer Joseph Thomson sold his wife, 'a born serpent', by auction.

Yet the law seldom considered the woman's view, and it was virtually impossible for a woman to dispose of a man. When Martha Robinson, beaten by her unstable husband who also infected her with gonorrhoea before trying to kill her by poison, sued for divorce in 1775, the judge instructed her to be more patient. And a century later, cold baths and enemas were still being swiftly instructed by doctors for women with involuntary thoughts about men.

The pervasive view of men was not just that women were inferior, but that being a woman constituted some sort of malady, especially after puberty. Menstruation was described in some medical texts as being a fault of women. Pain perceived by women was ascribed in some way to improper decorum. As late as 1892, a woman with cataracts was advised that only hysterectomy would restore vision.

▶ Women in medicine

At the Parthenon in Athens one day in 1850, a tiny owlet fell from its nest. The bird was spotted by a young woman who, sure it was about to be tortured to death by youths, shook them off and rescued it. She named the hatchling Athena, nursed it, hand-fed it and kept it safely in the pocket of her apron. The owl became her abiding companion. The woman's caring instincts would serve her well in her chosen career.

Women were excluded from medical training until the nineteenth century, before which their nursing and midwifery roles had been informal extensions of their mothering and domestic ones. Quite simply it was felt that women didn't have the constitution for medicine. The first female medical graduate appeared in 1849, Elizabeth Blackwell (1821–1910), top of her class at the Geneva Medical School in New York. The first woman in Britain to qualify was Elizabeth Garrett (1836–1917) in 1865 (officially, that is: in 1865 when British Army surgeon James Barry died, it was discovered that 'he' was a woman). Women were often excluded from the 'best' schools, and only after 1945 would women graduate from Yale or Harvard. Happily, by 1996, more women were graduating in Britain than men.

Nursing began its transformation in 1836 with the Deaconess Institute in Germany, founded to instruct young ladies to become nurse-deaconesses. Elizabeth Fry (1780–1845) visited it, before returning to London to found the Institute of Nursing in 1840. Shortly afterwards, a young Englishwoman named after her Florentine birthplace, Florence Nightingale (1820–1910), desperate to escape a stifled upbringing, visited, too. When shocking dispatches were sent from the Crimean War (1853–6) by *The Times* journalist W. H. Russell, where untrained male orderlies tended to wounded men in appalling conditions, Nightingale was moved to take 38 nurses to the barrack hospital at Scutari on the Black Sea. It was five years after she had rescued the owlet and Crimea was no place for a pet. Too domesticated to hunt, and family members failing to check on her in her attic, Athena perished while Nightingale prepared for her trip. Heartbroken, she delayed leaving for Scutari and found a taxidermist to preserve Athena forever.

At Scutari, Nightingale would transform everything. Mortality rates dropped from 40 per cent to 2 per cent within six months. The 'Lady with the Lamp' became so highly regarded that nurse training was formalized forthwith (1860) at St Thomas's Hospital. Nightingale's *Notes on Nursing* and *Notes on Hospitals* stressed hygiene, fresh air, strict discipline and devotion to the vocation. Her schools spread across continents to Australasia and North America where Dorothea Dix, Superintendent of the United States Army, had already made great strides in the American Civil War (1861–5).

▶ Maternity care and women's health

No doctor for most of history would perform a gynaecological examination, which explains why Mary Toft, a rabbit breeder from Guildford, for a number of weeks in 1726 was able to convince medical authorities that she was giving birth to rabbits. The sensation provoked King George I to send surgeons, including John Howard, 'eminent surgeon and man-midwife', to witness it. They were not disappointed, as she produced numerous rabbits (all dead) from beneath her garments.

Appreciation of almost anything gynaecological was still a long way off. A menstruating woman was often blamed for anything from poor harvests to killing off bees, and as late as 1878 the *British Medical Journal* ran a protracted column on whether her touch could 'spoil ham'. British doctors could be struck off the medical register for suggesting almost any gynaecological knowledge, whilst James Platt White in Buffalo, North America, was hounded by colleagues for allowing – with women's consent – childbirth to be observed.

Against these barriers, surgeon Isaac Baker Brown (1811–73) became a pioneering gynaecological surgeon, though with seriously deranged ideas. He was convinced that 'a large number of afflictions peculiar to females depended on loss of nerve power, produced by peripheral irritation, arising originally in some branches of the pudic nerve, more particularly the incident nerve supplying the clitoris'. In essence, he decided that women were unwell because they were continually masturbating, as suggested in his *The Curability of Certain Forms of Insanity, Epilepsy, Catalepsy, and Hysteria in Females*. His solution was to surgically remove – without their permission or prior knowledge – women's clitorises. He decided, too, that ovaries were better removed. His first three patients died. And so it was audacious that he should subject his fourth attempt on his sister, who lived, albeit with needlessly deranged body parts and fecundity. Baker Brown was thankfully expelled from the Obstetrical Society of London in 1867, and if there is a happy side to the story it is that his antics raised regard for women's anatomy.

Childbirth had long been viewed as a social, not medical, occasion. A physician in the 1700s would have said that medicine and midwifery had nothing in common. Midwifery was for uneducated females, and only rarely would a surgeon be asked to use some kind of instrument in obstructed labour. In 1827 a president of the Royal College of Physicians declared delivering babies 'foreign to the habits of a gentleman of enlarged academical education'. The Royal College of Surgeons rejected all association with midwifery. 'Nothing,' said one President, 'was more unnecessary or unmanly than for a surgeon or physician to neglect his patients, to sit by a lady's bedside for hours together in a natural labour which any female of prudence could manage.' Delivering babies was 'contrary to decency and common sense' said another. Any member found practising obstetrics surreptitiously was instantly expelled.

One American physician in 1852 said that 'women prefer to suffer the extremity of danger and pain rather than waive those scruples of delicacy which prevent their maladies from being fully explored'. Some doctors opposed forceps delivery on the grounds that it allowed women with small pelvises to bear children, thus passing on their inferiorities to daughters. Never mind that it often left those women dead.

But, bit by bit, surgeon-apothecaries (general practitioners) and 'man-midwives' or 'accoucheurs' (later, obstetricians) would become involved in labour. It was not until 1929 that the College of Obstetrics and Gynaecology was established, and until the early 1900s most deliveries were by untrained midwives, almost always at home. Some women with money favoured a nurse living in the home providing care around the time of childbirth and beyond. A general practitioner might deliver the baby, and take a fee.

That caesarean sections from the 1890s were not universally fatal must be regarded as progress. But the defeat of puerperal fever by sulfonamides, beginning just before World War II, remains the most important advance in the history of obstetrics. Antenatal and postnatal care would then become routine. By 1948 midwives (following three Acts) were providing organized, regulated maternity care, delivering most babies at home but with hospital deliveries on the rise. Yet many preventable deaths were not prevented. Some practitioners still disbelieved antisepsis, others finding the fee – 'a fraction of what the cabman would obtain for waiting at the gate' – dispiriting.

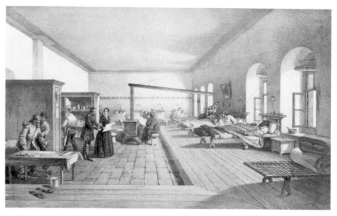

▲ Figure 12.1 Lithograph of Florence Nightingale's ward at Scatari by E Walker, 1908.

When the UK's National Health Service (NHS) was introduced, midwives, general practitioners and consultant obstetricians were poorly unified, but since labour can go alarmingly wrong alarmingly quickly, deliveries in maternity units steadily began to rise.

IV

The Ages of Modern Medicine: Twentieth-Century Medicine

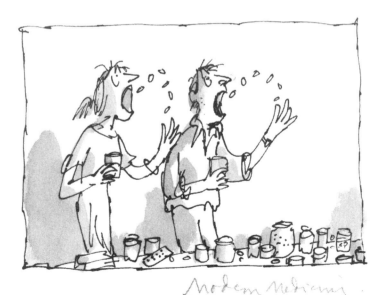

13

The Age of Pharmaceuticals

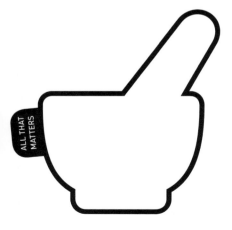

▶ Pharmaceutical beginnings

Until 1900, medical science had not translated into many effective therapies. Pharmacopoeias, largely herbal, were devised in antiquity. But until the 1800s most treatments were at best ineffective, frequently poisonous and often deadly. The only moderately effective drugs of the nineteenth century were opium for pain, quinine for malaria, colchicum for gout, digitalis to stimulate the heart and amyl nitrate to dilate the arteries in angina. The pharmaceutical box was still filled largely with blanks.

The twentieth century would change all that, a change that would be seeded in the tropics. Britain's expanding empire was impeded in this 'white man's grave', where mal-aria ('bad air') and other infections abounded, and so it is perhaps unsurprising that some of the earliest effective drugs would facilitate imperialism. Patrick Manson (1844–1922), Customs Medical Officer in Hong Kong in the 1870s, noticed how embryos of the tiny filarial worm, the cause of elephantiasis, were taken nocturnally from human blood by the *Culex* mosquito, developed in the insect and transmitted back to humans in bites: the first disease shown to be transmitted by an insect vector. Manson made tropical medicine an emergent specialty, later founding London's School of Tropical Medicine. Over the next generation it was found that schistosomiasis arose from a worm (its vector a snail), and amoebic dysentery from a nasty single-celled protozoan. Trypanosomiasis (sleeping sickness) was seen to be spread by flies. Malaria had been known since antiquity, and even in the nineteenth century 'marsh fever' could still be found in the fens of Cambridgeshire. It was British army surgeon Ronald Ross (1857–1932) who discovered the malarial parasite, happily thriving in the stomachs of *Anopheles* mosquitoes (only females) after biting his caged birds. Yellow fever was cracked next, linked to mosquitoes in Cuba; in 1900 bacteriologists James Carroll (1854–1907) and Jesse Lazear (1866-1900) would subject themselves experimentally to mosquito bites, fatally for Lazear.

The microbiological revolution launched by Pasteur and Koch had created interest in finding treatments (initially vaccines), the laboratory the crucible for a future medicine chest carrying live ammunition against disease.

Salvarsan for syphilis was one of the earliest effective antimicrobials. Mercury had been the potion of choice until the twentieth century, but there was reason to fear it – 'a night with Venus and a lifetime with Mercury', went the axiom – as bones degraded and teeth fell out. More importantly, it didn't work. But people were rightfully fearful of syphilis. It could lie dormant for years before erupting to provoke enduring misery. As well as sores, bone dissolution, heart disease and 'madness', noses frequently collapsed. London formed a 'No Nose'd Club' where people could 'show their scandalous vizards' without mockery. Sex, for centuries, had been appreciated as a means of contracting venereal disease, the term venereal having its etymology in 'Venus' the classical goddess of love, but microbial concepts of disease were only now being realized.

Microbiology, which fuelled some of the earliest effective drugs, would also fuel the new science of immunology. In 1884 Élie Metchnikoff (1845–1916) observed white blood cells overwhelming bacteria (phagocytosis), and developed the theory of host cells and antibodies fighting foreign antigens.

But, as it happened, it was chemical technology that would lead the way to therapeutics in the 1900s.

Pharmaceutical companies and research

Drugs could only be produced in meaningful quantities if there were places for production. Symbiosis between drug research and manufacture was needed, and in Germany and France chemical industries, established in the late 1800s, saw profit in diverting their interests towards the manufacture of drugs.

Emil von Behring (1854–1917) and Paul Ehrlich (1854–1915), two former assistants of Koch, had devised 'serum therapy' in which the serum of an animal rendered immune to tetanus or diphtheria by injection of attenuated bacteria (sufficient for the animal to produce antitoxin) could cure another exposed to an otherwise fatal dose of the bacteria. The first successful treatment was for a child with diphtheria in 1891. In Britain, Burroughs Wellcome & Co. would begin producing diphtheria antitoxin on a large scale and funding labs to pioneer more cures.

Ehrlich directed the Royal Prussian Institute for Experimental Therapy in Frankfurt-am-Main, financially supported by the commercial company that would become Hoechst. In 1905 he isolated *Treponema pallidum* as the cause of syphilis, in 1906 there was a diagnostic test and in 1907 over 600 arsenics were tried against it, Ehrlich taking out a patent for 606 – Salvarsan. Within three years Salvarsan had cured 10,000 people.

Attempts to find cures for other infections would prove disappointing for another 30 years, however, until Gerhard Domagk, research director of chemical company Bayer, discovered that a dye, Prontosil Red, appeared to treat mice infected with streptococci. He tested it on his daughter, conveniently suffering from erysipelas, saving her arm. Scientists at Paris's Pasteur Institute established that sulfanilamide (a sulfonamide component of the dye) was bacteriostatic, and it became readily and cheaply available (unable to be patented as it already existed). Immediately, puerperal fever rates declined, and in 1938 May and Baker developed M&B 693, a new 'sulfa' drug, more effective than sulfanilamide, that worked against a range of infections including erysipelas, mastoiditis, meningitis and gonorrhoea.

Pasteurian bacteriology would ultimately make biological, not chemical, therapies dominate future antimicrobial warfare. Folk wisdom taught that mouldy bread, applied to cuts, kept them clean (by the antibacterial action of fungi). Pasteur had noticed in 1877 that anthrax bacilli did not thrive when other bacteria were added. The notion that one creature destroys another to preserve its own life became known as antibiosis, the word 'antibiotic' (destroys life) later applied by soil microbiologist Selman Waksman.

Half a century later, in 1928, Alexander Fleming (1881–1955) and his wife Sarah were returning from an autumn holiday at their country retreat. Fleming, a Scottish bacteriologist at St Mary's Hospital, knew that harsh antiseptics applied to wounds were damaging, had already discovered the antibacterial enzyme lysozyme in tears and fluids, and now saw that mould had killed his staphylococcal colonies left in a Petri dish. For months he called the future penicillin 'mould-juice', which came from moulds of the genus *Penicillium*. He noted it killed many other bacteria, too. But mould-juice proved hard to reproduce, and was unstable. Ten years later Australian Howard Florey and Jewish-German émigré Ernst Chain in Oxford found that *Penicillium notatum* cured mice injected with streptococci. Pharmaceutical companies were preoccupied with wartime needs so, in 1941, he travelled to the United States to engineer production. When tested on wounded servicemen in North Africa in 1943 the results were phenomenal and within a year supplies were unlimited.

In 1945 Fleming, Florey and Chain shared a Nobel Prize.

▶ Pharmaceuticals

As research institute, university laboratory and industry collaborated, drugs went into mass production. Bayer marketed aspirin in 1900. Other antibiotics followed penicillin, including streptomycin and isoniazid for tuberculosis. The early 1900s also saw the notion of nutrition developing, and with the existence of vitamins proven (first mooted by Frederick Hopkins in Cambridge in 1912), manufacture could begin. Glaxo became a trademark for dried milk. Insulin was discovered by Frederick Banting and Charles Best in 1922 and used to convert a critical disease into a controllable one. Vaccines for diphtheria, whooping cough, tuberculosis, tetanus and yellow fever followed, tainted for a while by the Lübeck disaster when live tuberculosis bacillus contaminated the vaccine. Acetaminophen (paracetamol) appeared in 1948.

Many new drugs were set to appear after that.

By the 1950s fizzling sparklers had become exploding fireworks in the night sky of pharmaceutical endeavour.

14

The Age of Social Medicine and Diversification

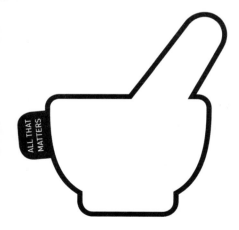

▶ Medicine and the state

In 1917 at Ruby Plains Station in the Kimberley, Western Australia, young stockman Jimmy Darcy fell from his horse and into a coma. He was transported to Hall's Creek, 40 miles away, where there was a telegraph station and a postmaster. The nearest doctor was half a continent away in Perth, called from his suburban practice to sit with a Morse operator, whereupon he diagnosed a ruptured bladder and advised immediate surgery. The postmaster would have to do it. Apprehensive at the prospect, without training and with just a razor and antiseptic, postmaster Tuckett was assured that Darcy's fate otherwise was certain death, something that did not alleviate his fears.

For seven hours, instructions relayed through telegraph wire, the postmaster persevered. What he did, incredibly, worked, and when Darcy died some days later the post-mortem examination, recounted by Reverend John Flynn (1880–1951), showed that an unrelated appendix abscess had weakened Darcy. It was concluded that the postmaster's efforts had been exemplary, but had there been remote clinics the abscess might have been detected earlier.

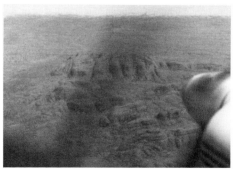

▲ Figure 14.1 Flying Doctor Service, Australia.

At the same time, and for the first time, war in Europe was being fought in the sky, prompting a young pilot to write to Flynn, who had developed nursing care for remote people, asking that if planes could be used in war, then why not in peace, to provide a medical service. Flynn committed himself to developing a national flying doctor network across Australia.

In the early twentieth century, medicine was still practised in largely disconnected ways (and in that sense Australia's Royal Flying Doctor Service was pioneering). Infections were being conquered. Sanitation had improved. But people – undernourished, toothless and lice-infested – were hardly 'healthy'. The state's role in health was ad hoc. Individual healthcare was a patchy mess of private, voluntary, religious and charitable practice. Professionals were becoming legally licensed, but ethics was a self-regulated area.

All this would change, continuously but unevenly, in the twentieth century. Prevention would need greater emphasis. 'Social medicine' would map disease, plotting it against income, education, class, diet and housing to highlight inequalities. Ideologies on national health issues ranged from the socialist left to the fascist right. Italy and Germany worshipped fitness, and saw it as a means to end all ills. Elsewhere, and in Britain in particular, the socialization of medicine (and later, to an extent, the 'medicalization' of society) took hold. The idea that the country would manage the health of its people, using scientific knowledge accrued in the preceding century, inspired great optimism.

▶ Dashed dreams and diversification

That optimism would be dashed by three devastating events in the first half of the twentieth century. The first would be World War I. The second would directly follow. The 1918

'Spanish flu' pandemic was unusually severe, spreading as far as the Arctic and Pacific, killing between 50 and 130 million people. The third would be World War II.

Notwithstanding these events, medicine developed and diversified apace. Wilhelm Röntgen (1845–1923) invented the X-ray in 1895 (though not the protective costumes later realized vital, and X-rays were taken liberally for diagnosis and endlessly for amusement). In 1900 Willem Einthoven (1860–1927) came up with electrocardiography. A year later the different human blood types were discovered. By 1921 epidural and local anaesthesia would be available. To prove it, that same year, Dr Evan Kane (1861–1932) performed an appendectomy on himself. To further prove his oddness, ten years later, aged 70, he nonchalantly disentangled his own inguinal hernia.

Surgery grew more daring, and was often needless. Sir William Arbuthnot-Lane (1856–1943) would remove yards of gut to treat constipation, and was so enraptured by his procedure that he urged it as a preventive measure. Lane's story is an unhappy one. A brilliant surgeon, his meeting with Russian bacteriologist Élie Metchnikoff in the early 1900s appears to have devastatingly influenced his thoughts. Lane had noticed that manual workers changed physically as a result of their work, leading him to consider that natural selection was happening much faster than Darwin had proposed. Metchnikoff had unfortunately become convinced of the same, and that several body parts were now obsolete and set to disappear. These included, Lane became convinced, the colon, which rather like the appendix was set to shrink and could one day be removed. Lane, unfortunately, had the expertise to remove colons, and began doing so with alarming enthusiasm. Despite being asked to lead the British army's surgical service during World War I, and setting up the first plastic and reconstructive surgery unit for war injuries, his reputation would become irreversibly damaged and he retired from medicine. London-based New Zealander Sir Harold Gillies (1882–1960), whose reputation opposed Lane's, pioneered wartime facial reconstructive surgery. He would also, much later, perform the first gender reassignment surgery. Lane's antics achieved renown. Yet soon afterwards, 20,000 brain lobotomies were performed in America, all needless. Tonsillectomies, adenoidectomies and hysterectomies would also become commonplace, mostly unnecessary.

By 1943 a dialysis machine had been invented and specialization in medicine was cementing. In the twentieth century, medical specialties – cardiology, respiratory medicine, gastroenterology, nephrology, neurology, endocrinology, haematology and oncology – would gradually crystallize. Surgery would branch out, too, into disciplines such as neurosurgery, vascular surgery and urology. Obstetrics and gynaecology and paediatrics were charting their own courses. Psychiatry would come into its own. Radiology would be a distinct discipline, as would an array of laboratory-based specialties. And public health medicine was set to rise.

War, as ever, spurred surgical advances. Sir Archibald McIndoe (1900–60) excelled in treating badly burned Royal Air Force crew of World War II. Antitoxins for tetanus and typhus stimulated pharmaceutical industry growth, and penicillin came just in time to treat many infected wounded.

But, alongside technical and therapeutic advances, this war would urgently demonstrate the need for an altogether new medical specialty.

▶ Experiments and ethics

In 1938 SS leader Heinrich Himmler sent an expedition to Tibet to find traces of a subterranean human race with 'vril' powers, and in time many Nazis would come to believe that

Aryans had descended from a 'vril' race. What most had forgotten, if they had ever known at all, was that the 'vril' people came not from subterranean Tibet, but from the imaginative mind of Edward Bulwer-Lytton, in whose 1871 science fiction novel *The Coming Race* they appear (in 1889 there would be sufficient recollection of them for *Bovril* to be named upon the notion that strength could be attained from hot water with bovine extract).

And so it was that Nazi Germany started its breeding programme to produce a 'master race'. It would be impossible for a writer today to recount the horrors of this period of history without diminishing what that account deserves, of how fellow humans were tortured, experimented on, gassed or 'burned whole' (the meaning of the word Holocaust). From a medical history perspective – the job of this book – we should soberly remind ourselves that 'mercy deaths' were 'legitimized', before the 'final solution' of the 'Jewish problem' was given full medical 'rationalization'. The complicity of German physicians and psychiatrists in this, on the basis that non-Aryans were defined as subhuman, allowed Mengele and others to do things we cannot begin to describe. And to murder six million people.

The Holocaust was not the first example of human experimentation. Episodes pervade history. Thousands were similarly killed at the South African concentration camp of Shark Island. In 1936 Shirō Ishii, a Japanese army microbiologist, exposed prisoners to anthrax and other deadly microbes. While the Tuskegee Syphilis Study, begun in the 1930s in Alabama, withheld penicillin from black Americans.

And throughout history medicine has grown its crop of murderers. Hawley Crippen poisoned his wife, burned her bones in the kitchen stove, dissolved her organs in acid and put her head in a handbag (thrown overboard on a day trip to France). John Adams was a much-loved general practitioner in Southend whose name kept appearing in the wills of deceased patients. He was arrested in 1956, by which time he was the richest doctor in England having killed, the Home Office believed, 163 people. And then there was Harold Shipman, an outwardly mild-mannered GP from Hyde in Yorkshire, who looked innocent to the last, perhaps because he looked a lot like Harrison Ford's Richard Kimble in *The Fugitive*. He killed over 250 people.

Of course these are appalling aberrations in the long and generally uplifting endeavours of medicine to help the human race. And though medical ethics formalized as a discipline followed the Nuremberg trials, it should be said that the subject is unendingly diverse, governing all practice and research, from day-to-day clinical decisions to research protocols to debates on genetic engineering.

15

The Age of 'Modern' Modern Medicine

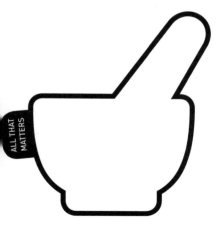

▶ Britain's NHS

Austerity, with rationing, defined a Britain re-equipping itself after war.

At the heart of what emerged from those years of hardship, however, was the National Health Service (NHS).

Between Disraeli's Public Health Act (1875) and World War I, British public health had gained momentum. Lloyd George's Liberal government (1906–14) provided school medical examinations and meals for underfed children, the National Insurance Act (1911) would protect workers in sickness, a principal contributor being socialist William Beveridge (1879–1963), and soon a Ministry of Health (1919) would be formed.

During World War II the government turned again to Beveridge for advice. A lawyer and economist, Beveridge had left politics for an academic career, firstly as Director of the London School of Economics (LSE) – where attempts to further eugenics ideas were relentlessly suppressed by the cheerfully and chivalrously named zoologist Lancelot Hogben – and thence Master of University College, Oxford. But his interest in social reform provided intellectual foundation for the NHS. Churchill thought Beveridge 'a windbag', but Churchill's coalition government asked Beveridge to look at how a post-war Britain might be built. Beveridge, predictably, considered this in immense detail, although it was an immense brief. *The Times* called the 1942 Beveridge Report *Social Insurance and Allied Services* 'a momentous document which should and must exercise a profound and immediate influence on the direction of social change in Britain'. The report chimed with public mood, outlining society's five giant evils – want, ignorance, disease, squalor and idleness – that needed to be overcome. It recommended a national system of social security in which compulsory payments would provide health and unemployment insurance, child benefit, maternity support and state pension. It also suggested a national health service.

Churchill's government tackled ignorance first, with the Education Act (1944), before Labour swept to power promising a 'cradle to grave' welfare state. Thus, Beveridge's main recommendations were implemented under Clement Attlee, to be funded from taxation, with the National Insurance and National Health Service Acts of 1946, the latter overseen by former miner and Minister of Health Aneurin ('Nye') Bevan. Within months, millions were enjoying false teeth, hearing aids and spectacles. Bevan called it 'the biggest single experiment in social service the world has ever undertaken', and would later reflect that it had 'become part of the texture of our national life. No political party would survive that tried to destroy it ... The essence of a satisfactory health service is that the rich and poor are treated alike, that poverty is not a disability, and wealth is not an advantage.'

Broadly similar developments occurred throughout Commonwealth nations, and across a Europe reeling from war a spectrum of state-aided welfare systems would grow, while America remained ideologically committed to private medicine.

▶ The contraceptive pill and the broader scope of medicine

In the post-war era came not just services for tackling disease, but development of interventions Beveridge and Bevan could have not envisaged. Perhaps the most influential was the oral contraceptive pill, approved by the US Food and Drug Agency in 1960.

It was followed, in juxtaposition, by an emergent field of reproductive medicine to aid infertile couples. The first beneficiary of in-vitro fertilization (IVF), in 1978, was Louise Brown, whose mother's fallopian tubes were blocked. Louise had a 'test-tube' baby sister in 1999. Just one. For sometimes IVF would do much more. Babies could be conceived in multiple, sometimes stupefying, numbers with reproductive technology, and sometimes staggeringly older women would experience childbirth. In 1992 a 61-year-old Italian woman would cause transient media frenzy for such an experience, before such an experience became more commonplace, tempered by ethical questions that did not have answers. Was it a human right to give birth at any age if technology made it possible? Was it right that a baby should be born to an aged mother or was that ageism? Many older parents argued that their life experience and ability to provide for a child was better than many younger parents.

In 1998, erections around the world became more robust and enduring with the introduction of sildenafil (Viagra®). Amid fierce debates about IVF, and a quarter of a century after liposuction started, Viagra® added to treatments that could not have been conceived at the NHS's inception.

Lifestyle-related health problems and an array of conditions that grey the boundaries of medicine, such as having too much hair (or too little), but for which treatment can improve quality of life, raised affordability questions. Perhaps nowhere more than in the field of medical aesthetics (by the twenty-first century over ten million cosmetic procedures were being performed annually in the United States), the era beyond pure cosmetic surgery in which, as well as reshaping noses and ears and vaginas, wrinkles, veins and every vexing blemish have a cure with needle, pill or laser.

By the end of the twentieth century, medicine's boundaries would be blurred.

But not before medicine had experienced a technological tornado.

▶ Technology

In 1967, US Surgeon General William Stewart famously declared: 'the time has come to close the book on infectious diseases. We have basically wiped out infection in the United States.' It seemed, at last, that medicine was winning the major battles against disease.

Medicine became increasingly integrated in the second half of the twentieth century. Institutions – hospitals, laboratories and universities – collaborated. And medical science could make the fastest progress in history. The expanse of knowledge and its application was relentless, and we can but point out drops in that sea of advancement. In those 50 years, technology doubtless had the greatest impact.

Technology revolutionized diagnosis. It converted laboratories from dusty desktops of Petri dishes to capacious suites of diagnostic capability. Chemical analysis of blood, microbiological testing, immunological investigation and examination of pathological specimens all started going on feverishly behind the scenes in which clinicians operated. New radiological methods appeared: ultrasound in the 1950s, and computed tomography (CT) in the 1970s, followed hotly by magnetic resonance imaging (MRI), positron emission tomography (PET) and a wide range of nuclear techniques, all with diversifying modes of operation to identify almost whatever seemed necessary to identify. MRI could be adjusted depending upon the density of tissue being examined, to examine different aspects of brain matter or cartilage in a knee. Nuclear medicine could employ all manner of (safe) radioactive particles to highlight body structures. And fibre optic technology made it possible to peer into areas of body previously inaccessible, and treat disease without resorting to major surgery.

Technology revolutionized treatment, with new drugs and devices. Pharmaceutical companies had matured from dabbling in antimicrobial production to producing hundreds of antibiotics and thousands of other drugs. The number of pills for heart disease shook pockets like a rattlesnake. Drugs for chest conditions could be inhaled. Skin problems had ointments and creams. Psychiatry entered its new era with Prozac®. New, more potent, antibacterial antibiotics came about, and anti-viral drugs arrived. And unexpected things happened. In 1984 two Australians, Barry Marshall and Robin Warren, reported that *Helicobacter pylori* bacteria, once thought specks of dirt under microscopes, were nasty little organisms that caused stomach ulcers. Soon antibiotics for ulcers made surgery for ulcers a rarity. And at the interface with surgery, anti-rejection drugs allowed organ transplantation to flourish.

New drugs are only part of the story in disease intervention. 'Interventional' techniques took medicine and surgery from mere removal of upset organs to restoration of function: in the 1940s dialysis; in 1949 the intraocular lens; in 1952 open heart and valve surgery; in 1954 kidney transplantation; in 1959 the cardiac pacemaker; in 1962 hip replacement; in 1963 liver and lung transplantation; in 1967 heart transplantation; in 1969 cochlear implantation; in 1981 heart-lung combined transplantation; and in 1985 robots began to play alongside human surgeons in operating on humans. Artificial joints are now implanted routinely in hips and knees severely damaged by arthritis. Video monitors and laparoscopic instruments routinely permit removal of gall bladders through a few small incisions. Radiologists now routinely treat disease from the end of exploratory instruments whose journeys are made possible by technology. Technology has made more treatment possible. And clinicians have developed new skills to use technology.

And technology revolutionized prevention. Immunization continued its advance with modern vaccines: in 1955 Salk for polio; in 1962 Sabin for oral polio (vaccine-laced sugar cubes); in 1964 for measles; in 1967 for mumps; in 1970 for rubella; in 1980 for hepatitis B; and in 1992 for hepatitis A. Outbreaks of botulism, a food-borne disease produced by one of the deadliest known toxins producing paralysis, led researchers to muse about turning that toxin into a useful drug for serious neurological problems where paralysing specific muscles would help. That vision became Botox®, whose most common use would become the temporary erasing of wrinkles.

Medicine advanced in the late twentieth century more than in all of earlier history. So much happened that it is often difficult, unlike in earlier years, to credit any endeavour to one individual. Advances were collaborative, and incremental. As geneticist Steve Jones said, in science it is easier to be 'mediocre' and make a difference, meaning that while perhaps in art only the more superlative creations find success, a modest stitch in science's immodest tapestry forms an integral part.

Yet for all that we learned in that last half-century, we were ignorant of far more. The gains brought new challenges. William Stewart's comment was premature indeed, as almost immediately microbes proved they could transform and resist antibiotics. Ever more lethal strains appeared with alacrity and ease. And altogether new ones appeared to greet us with glee. Lassa fever, a haemorrhagic viral infection, appeared in 1969, isolated from a missionary nurse who flew to New York City from Nigeria. The equally deadly Marburg and Ebola viruses followed. Others, like West Nile fever, have moved from one area of the world to another. For decades, the West Nile virus caused outbreaks in Africa and Europe; in 1999 it appeared in New York, from whence it spread quickly through North America. Eradication of smallpox shortened the list of diseases by one, the only naturally occurring disease humans have ever wiped out. Its last fatal case was in 1978, just before the human immunodeficiency virus (HIV) would introduce itself to the world.

The fight against infection sees both sides – technology and disease – head-locked in fierce development of novel moves to try to thwart the other.

Advancement and disappointment are often hand in hand.

No more so than in two other scourges of our modern world: heart disease and cancer.

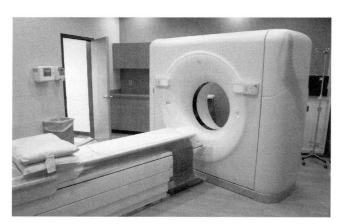

▲ Figure 15.1 Modern medical technology.

16

The Age of Today

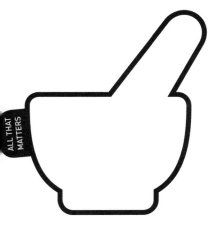

▶ The twin spectres of heart disease and cancer

When President Dwight Eisenhower suffered a heart attack in the middle of the night on 24 September 1955, his physician told Mamie Eisenhower to snuggle with her husband in bed and keep him warm. Eisenhower was given morphine for pain, and allowed to sleep until noon before a cardiologist was called to perform an electrocardiogram (ECG). Later, the president went to hospital by car, where he was confined to seven weeks of bed-rest.

On 27 October 2008, Professor Eugene Braunwald, one of the world's most engaging cardiologists, gave a lecture to the Royal College of Physicians in London entitled *Emerging Insights into Antiplatelet Therapy*. It had long been known that heart attacks occurred when atheromatous deposits in the heart's arteries cracked, releasing chemical messengers alerting the body to injury. The body's response to any injury – causing blood to clot – has been unchanged through evolution, evolution that has not adjusted to modern perils such as atheroma. A blood clot is the first thing prehistorically mustered in injury, yet the last thing a heart needs. Braunwald's lecture eloquently united the many thousands of therapeutic developments that had occurred in the fifty years from Eisenhower's heart attack to inhibit platelets, the blood cells integral to clots forming.

Surgical advances predated pharmacological ones in cardiology. Open-heart surgery was pioneered as early as the 1940s, closing holes between chambers and manipulating valves. The next big advance, in 1958, was the pacemaker to counteract a slow heart rate. A positively electrifying moment came in the early 1960s when Bernard Lown of Harvard reported how a shock of direct current applied to the chest could safely correct dangerous heart rhythms. It paved the way for modern defibrillation and cardiopulmonary resuscitation (CPR). And then in 1967 Christiaan Barnard performed his famous first human heart transplantation. Human kidney transplantation had already proved successful – although in 1963 surgeons transplanted chimpanzee kidneys into humans with, they had happily reported, technical success (all patients subsequently died) – and so when 23-year-old Denise Darvall died after a traffic accident, Barnard sewed her heart into the chest of 54-year-old Louis Washkansky. Washkansky died of pneumonia 18 days later, but Barnard's second patient lived for 18 months. Unhappily new practices in medicine, when first applied to humans, even after the lengthy research, often have a learning curve. Brief regression in outcomes may be seen before progress.

That was the challenge with cardiac stents. Angioplasty, the procedure to clear arteries, was in the 1990s gradually being superseded by stent devices to keep vessels open. Stents were initially regarded with scepticism – not least by surgeons now comfortable with bypass surgery – but within a decade stenting became the commonest intervention for blocked coronary arteries.

When Eisenhower had his heart attack, heart disease was the main killer in the West, and so it remains. But many more deaths would occur without these advances. As well as drugs to dissolve clots, statins may be given to lower cholesterol, an array of pills to lower blood pressure, beta-blockers to lower heart rate and agents to block the body's angiotensin system, a system of hormones erroneously activated by the kidney which perceives its reduced blood supply as due to blood loss, not a failing heart, promoting fluid retention, something which only adds to the strain on the heart. Diuretics can eliminate unwanted body fluid, and treatments for heart failure continue to arrive apace. And now implanted devices can serve as both pacemakers and defibrillators to automatically detect a life-threatening abnormal rhythm and shock the heart out of it.

Stroke continues its relentless rise in the modern world, too. Equally unanticipated by evolution, the brain's modest blood supply is ill-equipped for the vascular damage brought by modern lifestyles, such that minor faults sometimes provoke devastating clinical earthquakes if vital brain territory is blood-deprived.

Heart disease and cancer became in the twentieth century the major causes of morbidity and mortality as infectious diseases were at least quieted, if not quelled, and the world wars were over. People started to live longer lives, attributable to improved living standards and better healthcare. Suddenly, it was appreciated that a double-edged sword of living longer was development of diseases hitherto less common, including cancers associated with greater exposure to the 'stuff of life' with human organs increasingly susceptible to genetic mutations and faulty programming.

Just after World War II pharmacologists Louis Goodman and Alfred Gilman had noted that in mustard-gas victims lymph tissue (which grows cancerously in lymphoma) was suppressed. They tested it and other agents on mice with lymphoma, and while their 'treatments' were also 'poisons', the notion of a drug in the right quantity to 'poison' rapidly dividing cancer cells at a greater rate than normal cells would lead the way to modern chemotherapy in cancer, alongside ever-improving surgical techniques and radiotherapy.

Inarguably more effective in the fight against cancer is screening to detect and treat early disease. And debatably more effective than any current therapies are those arising from the sciences of genetics and immunology.

▶ The twin promises of genetics and immunology

In the 1950s two unknown academics at King's College, London, were musing about molecules. The New Zealand-born Maurice Wilkins (1916–2004) was reservedly disposed, and had spent much of the war helping design the atomic bomb. Rosalind Franklin (1920–58) was less retiring, often forthright, and a bit of an enigma. What studying science meant to her was relayed in a letter by the 20-year-old to her father: 'science and everyday life cannot and should not be separated. Science, for me, gives a partial explanation of life ...' Those words would presage something Franklin would later discover, of perhaps unparalleled magnitude to science before or since.

It was an unlikely quartet of scientists in England, two in Cambridge and two at King's, who would decipher DNA. Unlikely, because as well as being novices – Franklin and Wilkins arguably less so than James D. Watson (1928–) and Francis Crick (1916–2004) – they seldom got on. The most unlikely was Watson, an American genius and keen bird-watcher who had entered University aged fifteen. In 1951, he was a confident 23-year-old at the Cavendish Laboratory in Cambridge who appeared to enjoy most things over work. Crick, twelve years older and without a doctorate, was indisputably more 'academic', impatient and, by most accounts, socially less at ease. Neither Watson nor Crick was trained in biochemistry. As Watson cheerfully remarked in his book *The Double Helix* (1968), 'it was my hope that the gene might be solved without my learning any chemistry'.

There is little doubt that Franklin could be intransigent, to the point and seldom diplomatic. In *The Double Helix* she is depicted as secretive and deliberately unsexy: 'though her features were strong, she was not unattractive and might have been quite stunning had she taken even a mild interest in clothes. This she did not. There was never lipstick to contrast with her straight black hair, while at the age of thirty-one her dresses showed all the imagination of English blue-stocking adolescents.' In the book, whose aim was to describe the unravelling of DNA, much time is spent musing over the bad-tempered 'Rosy' who hoarded her data and might have been pretty had she taken off her glasses and done something with her hair. It would seem too obvious to suggest that Watson fancied her, but he probably did.

Or that he envied her knowledge. 'Rosy' – a name to which she had never responded – had the best images anywhere of the possible structure of DNA, achieved through the technique of X-ray crystallography allowing atoms and molecules to be visualized. It had been used to map atoms in crystals (hence the name), but DNA molecules were much more recalcitrant, and only Franklin was getting good results. Indeed Franklin, rather a perfectionist, had exquisite results. She was the first to recognize phosphorus atoms in the helix, proving these to be on the outside and the helix to be double, unlike the interpretation of Linus Pauling, America's leading chemist of the time.

Franklin, it must be said, was not forthcoming with her findings – to Wilkins' exasperation and Watson and Crick's exploitation – and cannot be altogether blamed. Female academics in the 1950s were treated with disdain. 'I'm afraid we always used to adopt – let's say a patronizing attitude towards her', Crick later recalled. In the summer of 1952, Franklin oddly did something that would provoke antipathy in Wilkins and extinguish any chance of her being credited with the helix's structure. To Wilkins' chagrin, she posted a mock notice around King's announcing the death of the DNA helix. The outcome was that in January 1953 Wilkins showed Watson Franklin's images, 'apparently without her knowledge or consent'.

Years later, Watson would concede that this 'was the key event' that gave him and Crick impetus to succeed. It was known that DNA had four components – adenine, guanine, cytosine and thymine – pairing up in specific ways. By playing with pencil-sketches and pieces of cardboard cut into molecules, Watson and Crick were able to work out how these fitted together. They made a model of DNA: a double helix, right-handed with the two strands running in opposite directions. It was inarguably brilliant work, with or without Franklin's 'help', and on 25 April 1953, *Nature* carried the 900-word article by Watson and Crick 'A Structure for Deoxyribose Nucleic Acid'.

Rosalind Franklin died of ovarian cancer, aged just 37, four years before the Nobel Prize was awarded to Watson and Crick. Her part in history has now been largely redressed, and the science of genetics has galloped on swiftly.

In 1859 Charles Darwin (1809–82) published *On the Origin of Species* (noting different insects on holiday in Wales to those in his native Shrewsbury, long before joining *HMS Beagle*) and in 1866 Gregor Mendel (1822–84) on modes of inheritance. Darwin concluded that diversity was vital, which questions the extent to which we should interfere with natural diversification processes.

Genetic manipulation is not new. Genetically modified organisms have been created for decades. Bacteria can be genetically engineered to contain human sequences of DNA to produce, as they multiply, large quantities of human proteins such as insulin. Polymerase chain reaction (PCR) technology, which amplifies DNA sequences, has broad diagnostic applications, while DNA profiling has changed the face of forensic work and profiling the human genome provokes debate about predicting diseases. Stem cell research continues inexhaustibly. A stem cell is an early 'generic' cell that has the ability to produce 'specific' cells, such as heart or brain cells. Stem cells from cloned embryos can potentially create new tissues or organs, but the creation of embryos for research and therapeutics engenders fierce ethical debate. Cloning organisms is easily possible: Dolly the sheep became the world's first cloned animal in 1999. Food shortages for a bulging population may be alleviated by genetically modifying foods, creating crops resistant to disease or drought. But unwittingly we might create organisms causing extinction of others by out-competing or carrying lethal disease. And science now has the wherewithal to genetically engineer a woolly mammoth. But would it be kind to produce one (almost certainly not just one) and what ecological damage might there be to interfering with nature?

Against this, the role of medicine has almost always been to interfere with the processes of nature. In 1981 a new disease that was sweeping the world, acquired immune deficiency syndrome (AIDS) caused by HIV, demanded that medicine respond rapidly to do just that. HIV, which parasitizes the human immune system, drove medical science to explore the eloquent workings of the immune system and understanding where HIV made it faulty. Treatments led to the virus mutating and again medical science found itself in a war of ingenuity with an organism that could disarmingly rearm itself through genetic restructuring. Prognosis is now vastly improved, largely through combination treatments which suppress the virus's ability to mutate, but maintaining this status quo requires patients to adhere strictly to treatment regimens, something not easy to enforce, particularly in resource-poor areas where treatment availability may be limited. HIV infection, perhaps more than any disease, highlights global inequalities in healthcare.

We can now more effectively treat more diseases, but there are now more diseases to treat. Whereas HIV infection is the most notable immune-deficiency disease, many diseases, such as rheumatoid arthritis, arise through over-exuberance of immunological mechanisms leading to inflammation. Traditional drugs to dampen down inflammation carry many side-effects, and therapies that inhibit molecules within aberrantly activated immune signalling chains may be the way forward for many diseases. Molecular therapies are finding their place, too, in switching off signalling pathways in cancers that allow cells to divide.

Molecular therapies almost defined the close of the twentieth century.

And at the close of that century genetics and molecular biology took a new direction of interest. As people got older, scientists became curious as to how they aged.

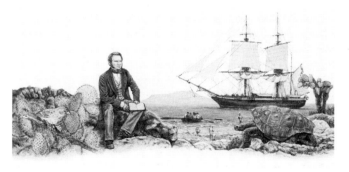

▲ Figure 16.1 Charles Darwin, Galápagos.

▶ The twin dilemmas of obesity and ageing

Life expectancy is an intriguing thing. All species have their own anticipated time on earth. Some koi reportedly live 200 years. Bowhead whales may live to 200, making them the oldest mammals. One of Darwin's Galápagos tortoises, Harriet, died in 2006 aged 175. Conversely, the lifespan of a mayfly can be 30 minutes and is seldom more than a day.

Humans fit somewhere in between. Females consistently outlive males. The longest living human was Jeanne Calment of France, who died in 1997 at the age of 122 years, 164 days. She met van Gogh in 1888 when he bought paint and pencils from her father's shop; she described him as dirty, badly dressed and disagreeable. She watched the Eiffel Tower being built. At 85 she took up fencing and at 100 rode a bicycle. She was otherwise inspiringly unathletic and ascribed her longevity to olive oil, port and around a kilogram of chocolate a week.

Two healthcare problems of the Western world incontestably pose today's biggest challenges: obesity (and concomitant type 2 diabetes), rates of which are unprecedented; and ageing (although if obesity and diabetes continue the latter will cease).

A world of better health and social care, at least in the West, with its demographic of older people, poses difficult questions. Society must decide its healthcare priorities, and ethics ensure that older people are not prejudiced.

In 2007, researchers at the Salk Institute for Biological Studies, California, identified a gene in worms linking eating less with living longer. There has long been debate about whether low ingestion enhances longevity in humans, but research suggests that relative fasting reduces growth factors responsible for accelerating the risk of heart disease, cancer and dementia.

And it seems that active people who walk each day live as long as those with exuberant enthusiasm for activity (although much longer than those who do nothing).

All evidence supports a life of all things in moderation.

Pretty much a life that Jeanne Calment lived.

Postscript

Today disquiet pervades medicine. The mid-twentieth century's optimism has waned. Excitement bubbled over penicillin, heart transplantation and test-tube babies. Now the effervescence has gone, with, for example, growing antibiotic resistance, fears around biotechnology, and realization of medicine's limitations. At the same time, health costs soar. The UK's NHS may disintegrate. Insurance costs and litigation claims dog medicine. In rich countries, many needy people get poor treatment. In developing countries, most are in need; tropical diseases remain rampant, while war, poverty and famine thwart basic healthcare provision.

Medicine's difficulties are partly the price of progress. In the old days things were simple. People had lower expectations and seldom complained. Medicine's job was to lessen lethal disease and relieve suffering. But then its goals became less clear. Where the job of tackling disease was being done, was medicine to become a service industry to provide for 'clients' with their own notions about health and lifestyle enhancement? Ironically, the healthier society gets, the more medicine it craves, especially in the United States where free market pressures are created by medical profession, business and media. Scares about new conditions arise. People are urged into more tests and ever more conditions are revealed. Expensive treatments are offered. A clinician choosing not to investigate or treat is open to malpractice. Should governments devote more public money to public health? Jenner's work on vaccination in the eighteenth century, Snow's epidemiological work on cholera in the nineteenth, and Doll and Hill's landmark work on smoking's association with cancer in the twentieth emphasized the place of preventive medicine.

But now, amid rising expectations, the service industry of medicine is struggling again to meet the basic demands of managing lethal disease and relieving suffering. People are getting older. And there are a lot more people. Debates about rationing continue, about who may qualify for expensive drugs and whether or not a public-funded health service should fund 'self-inflicted' conditions. The age of the Internet has revolutionized medicine. But it has also opened the door for illicit activity, such as illicit marketing of substances.

The doubling of the world's population in the 50 years from 1950 to 2000, a population now over 7 billion, has in no small part been helped by medical intervention. The contraceptive pill, in theory at least, paved the way for a means to control that population.

We now stand on the precipice of the future, not knowing what it holds. But if the early years of the 21st century are anything to go by, and if we think instead about what is good, we can look forward to continuous improvements. In 2005, we saw the first partial face transplant. In 2008 a full face appeared. Newer stents reduced the risk of coronary arteries occluding. Gene therapy offers promise. Molecular therapies pop up like bluebells to treat disease. HIV shifted from being an inexorably fatal disease to a manageable chronic one. Evidence tells us more than ever how to best treat disease. More disease than ever is prevented. Human papilloma virus vaccination will prevent most cases of cervical cancer. Smoking cessation battles are being won. And a patient education revolution, aided by the Internet, means that never before have patients been so empowered to participate in their health. And when, in 2003, a new disease, severe acute respiratory syndrome, spread around the world, collaborative international effort rapidly stemmed the outbreak.

We should take comfort that we have come a long way. We no longer burn people as witches. We no longer laugh at mental illness (generally). We no longer treat heart attacks at home. We have cures for infections. We have advanced surgery. We have impressive diagnostics and effective treatments for heart disease and cancer and thousands of diseases in between. Our world cares more for fellow humans than perhaps ever in history (even if it doesn't always seem that way). And we have wisdom, intelligence, resilience and hope.

And, as Darwin revealed, an ability to survive.

30 dates providing historical context to events in this book

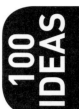

1. 11000–6000 BC: Neolithic Revolution.
2. 3500 BC: Egyptian civilization begins.
3. 750 BC–330 AD: Ancient Greece.
4. 79: Vesuvius erupts (Pliny the Elder dies; Pliny the Younger recounts it).
5. 500: Middle Ages begin.
6. 800: Charlemagne, Frankish king, crowned.
7. 911: Viking leader Rollo granted land in Normandy for Charles the Simple remaining English king.
8. 1016: Ethelred the Unready finally succumbs to Danish reprisals and Cnut's takeover.
9. 1066: William the Conqueror's Normans (North or Norsemen) defeat Harold II at Hastings.
10. 1066: French to become language of the English Court for 300 years.
11. 1096: The Crusades begin.
12. 1305: Renaissance art begins.
13. 1473: First book printed in English, *Recuyell of the Historyes of Troye*.
14. 1492: Columbus reaches the Americas (but it is explorer Amerigo Vespucci after whom America is named).
15. 1485–1603: The Tudors, beginning with Henry VII, ending with Elizabeth I's death, succeeded by James I.
16. 1536: Beheading of Anne Boleyn, accused of adultery and witchcraft for having three nipples (one a mole).
17. 1588: Spanish Armada's defeat.
18. 1600: British East India Company founded, followed by Dutch and French equivalents.
19. 1620: The *Mayflower* Pilgrim Fathers leave Plymouth to found America.
20. 1649: Charles I executed during the English Civil War between Royalists and Oliver Cromwell's Parliamentarians.
21. 1660: Charles II's Restoration (later, successor James II flees as William of Orange lands in England).
22. 1775–83: The American Revolution.
23. 1788: Captain James Cook arrives in New South Wales.
24. 1789: George Washington becomes first president of the United States.
25. 1789: The French Revolution, leading Antoine Lavoisier, pioneer of modern chemistry, to the guillotine.
26. 1805: Battle of Trafalgar, Admiral Lord Nelson defeating the French.
27. 1815: Battle of Waterloo, the Duke of Wellington defeating Napoleon's French.

28. 1831–36: Charles Darwin's *HMS Beagle* voyage.
29. 1853–56: Crimean War.
30. 1861–65: American Civil War, culminating in the end of slavery in the United States.

10 facts about the history of medicine

31. History of medicine began as an academic discipline in Leipzig, under Karl Sudhoff (1853–1938).
32. Sudhoff was succeeded by Henry Sigerist (1891–1957) in 1925.
33. Sigerist went to impart the subject in America as Germany became Nazist.
34. Charles Singer (1876–1960) was Britain's first historian of medicine, at University College London (UCL).
35. Sir Henry Wellcome (1853–1936) bequeathed vast capital for a medical charity, and his artefact collection.
36. It included skulls, a Peruvian mummy, Napoleon's toothbrush and George III's hair.
37. Wellcome's trustees chose UCL as the Wellcome Trust's home.
38. The later Wellcome Institute comprised Museum and Library, and later the Wellcome Collection.
39. It was praised by a certain James Watson, disparaging America's lack of science museums.
40. America does, in truth, have plentiful science museums, and Watson found his place in them with his rather feebly named collaborator Crick, who far from feebly announced outside Cambridge's Eagle pub in 1953, 'we have discovered the secret of life'.

10 places to explore medical history

41. The Wellcome Collection.
42. The Royal College of Surgeons' Hunterian Museum, London, for those intrigued by anatomical 'fauna'.
43. The British Museum (and Director Neil MacGregor's *A History of the World in 100 Objects*).
44. The Florence Nightingale Museum, also home to her stuffed owl, Athena.
45. Edward Jenner's Museum, Berkeley, where he enjoyed marriage to Catherine, fossils and grapevines.
46. The Alexander Fleming Laboratory Museum, London, where his laboratory is restored to its 1928 condition.
47. The National Museum of Health and Medicine, Maryland, holding 25 million artefacts (including Einstein's brain).
48. The Pasteur Institute, Paris.
49. Roy Porter's *The Cambridge History of Medicine* and *Blood and Guts*.
50. Douglas Guthrie's dated (1945) but deft history of medicine.

10 facts about medicine and art

51. Prehistoric cave art depicts ritual dances.
52. Ancient pots depict physicians examining patients.
53. Medieval art was often dominated by images of plague.
54. Renaissance artists captured, consciously and unconsciously, pathological signs.
55. Renaissance artists also began illustrating for education, producing elaborate anatomy atlases.
56. Models in some Rubens (1577–1640) paintings appear to have breast cancer.
57. Animals began appearing in medical art for perspective. Clara ate at the dinner table with the East India Company director, before coming to Europe in 1741. Evolution has seen aquatic, pygmy and woolly rhinos. Clara was an Indian rhino, a first in medical art.
58. C. J. Staniland (1838–1916) painted with such detail and mood that it cannot be said that nothing interesting ever came out of his hometown Hull (though it is true that nothing interesting has ever happened in Hull).
59. For *The Doctor*, Luke Fildes (1843–1927) drew on the death of his eldest son.
60. Sir Quentin Blake's 'As Large as Life' exhibition for hospitals included *Ordinary Life*, celebrating everyday life with characters picnicking, picking apples and feeding birds, and *Mothers and Babies Underwater*.

10 facts about medicine and literature

61. Greek classics describe illness.
62. Hippocratic writings were the first to dispel magic.
63. Syphilis features liberally in Shakespeare, Dickens and Voltaire.
64. Vesalius's *On the Workings of the Human Body* (1543) revolutionized medicine.
65. Plague was the basis for Daniel Defoe's *A Journal of the Plague Year*. His *Robinson Crusoe* was the first English novel.
66. The most famous literary doctor is perhaps Sir Arthur Conan Doyle's John H. Watson.
67. Doctors pop up where the story itself isn't medical, as in Charlotte Brontë's *Jane Eyre* and Jane Austen's *Sense and Sensibility*.
68. Samantha Harvey's *The Wilderness* describes the mind's descent into dementia, and its effects on those around the sufferer.
69. Oliver Sacks recounted many fascinating cases.
70. Novelists are often doctors or health professionals, such as Somerset Maugham, A. J. Cronin and Michael Crichton.

5 examples of medicine on screen

71. Dr Kildare.
72. M*A*S*H.

73. Quincy.
74. E.R.
75. House.

5 facts about animals in medicine

76. Animals permitted farming, and so civilization.
77. Animals, albeit without consent, add to medical science through experimentation.
78. Animals provide therapeutic drugs, from the early days of insulin to novel drugs from the seabed.
79. Animals enhance people's life expectancy: from eating fish to owning a dog.
80. Animals enrich our lives (like Sir David Attenborough).

5 ways to increase life expectancy

81. Move more (spend more time outside).
82. Eat less.
83. Be married (to the right person).
84. Have friends.
85. Own a dog.

5 ways to decrease life expectancy

86. Move less (spend more time watching television).
87. Eat more.
88. Be married (to the wrong person).
89. Have enemies.
90. Own a wolf.

5 types of nurse

91. Matron (senior nurse in managerial role).
92. Staff nurse (trained nurse).
93. Specialist nurse (nurse in specialized role).
94. Healthcare assistant (untrained nurse).
95. Nurse shark (inshore bottom-dwelling cartilaginous fish – swims around a bit, but ineffective in patient care).

5 distorters of medical truths

96. Nutritionists (not to be confused with dietitians; dietitians are professionals, nutritionists self-appointed).
97. The *Daily Mail*.
98. The media generally.
99. Alternative practitioners (some)
100. Politicians (all).

Meet the Author

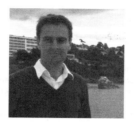

Tim Hall, MBChB (Aberdeen), FRCP (London), MRCGP, DipClinEd, FHEA, graduated as a doctor from Aberdeen University Medical School. He spent many years living in Australia, working in remote Aboriginal communities as well as Perth and Fremantle. He is a Fellow of the Royal College of Physicians and author of textbooks for junior doctors. He is naturally curious about the world. His favourite things include beaches, Devon and Cornwall, animals, people (well, some people), history and just about anything that is fascinating or funny. He is thrilled and enormously grateful that his (indeed the world's) favourite artist, Sir Quentin Blake, chose to collaborate with this book.

Acknowledgements

I am enormously grateful to Sir Quentin Blake for his kind gift, to me, of original illustrations for this book. A proportion of money I receive from its sales will go to medical charities.

I greatly appreciate the hard work done by Hodder - Sam Richardson my editor, Helen Rogers, Gareth Haman and all working for the Hodder team.

Huge thanks, of course, goes to my agent and friend, Frances Kelly. Her energy, enthusiasm and expertise, and her enduringly caring spirit for the book and its author, have been steadfast.

Image Credits

Chapter 1 Swimming reindeer © The Trustees of the British Museum. **Chapter 2** Egyptian clay cattle © The Trustees of the British Museum. **Chapter 3** Roman baths © Ran Dembo/ Shutterstock. **Chapter 4** River Avon © pjhpix/Shutterstock. **Chapter 8** Edward Jenner's home © Courtesy of the Jenner Museum. **Chapter 12** A Ward in the Hospital at Scutari, engraved by E. Walker, 1856 (colour litho), Simpson, William 'Crimea' (1823-99)/Florence Nightingale Museum, London, UK/The Bridgeman Art Library. **Chapter 14** Royal Flying Doctor Service © Tim Hall. **Chapter 15** Medical technology © SNEHIT/Shutterstock. **Chapter 16** Charles Darwin © Dorling Kindersley/Thinkstock.

All artwork by Sir Quentin Blake: permission of A P Watt at United Agents on behalf of Quentin Blake.

Index